Augmentative and Alternative Communication

Models and Applications for Educators, Speech–Language Pathologists, Psychologists, Caregivers, and Users

Augmentative and Alternative Communication

Models and Applications for Educators, Speech–Language Pathologists, Psychologists, Caregivers, and Users

Filip Loncke, PhD

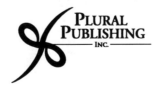

PLURAL
PUBLISHING
INC.

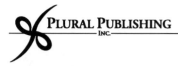

5521 Ruffin Road
San Diego, CA 92123

e-mail: info@pluralpublishing.com
Website: http://www.pluralpublishing.com

Typeset in 10.5/13 Palatino by Flanagan's Publishing Services, Inc.
Printed in the United States of America by McNaughton & Gunn, Inc.
19 18 17 16   2 3 4 5

Library of Congress Cataloging-in-Publication Data

Loncke, Filip, author.
  Augmentative and alternative communication : models and applications for educators, speech-language pathologists, psychologists, caregivers, and users / Filip Loncke.
      p. ; cm.
  Includes bibliographical references and index.
  ISBN-13: 978-1-59756-498-4 (alk. paper)
  ISBN-10: 1-59756-498-2 (alk. paper)
  I. Title.
  [DNLM: 1. Communication Aids for Disabled. 2. Communication Disorders—rehabilitation. 3. Interpersonal Relations. 4. Linguistics. 5. Needs Assessment. 6. Nonverbal Communication. WL 340.2]
  RC423
  616.85'503—dc23
                                              2013047557

Contents

Introduction

Human communication is amazing. It is fast, it is well-organized (and complicated), and it can take on many forms (it is flexible). Augmentative and alternative communication (AAC) is a testimony of the resilience of the human capacity to communicate, as well as of the natural tendency to adapt and adjust when typical forms of communication are not working as well. AAC is the field that describes and explains the methods, tools, and theories of the use of nonstandard linguistic and nonlinguistic communication by and with individuals without or with limited functional speech (see Chapter 1).

Today, AAC is used by an ever-growing group of individuals of all ages, each with their own personal and communication needs. For communication, some people use gestures or manual signs, while others use graphic symbols to get their messages across. Today many AAC users operate speech-generating devices, and everyday there are more who use smart phones or electronic tablets (McNaughton & Light, 2013).

This book is an attempt to describe AAC comprehensively and to offer a framework that helps to understand what AAC intervention does (and does not) in the process of communication. Some AAC interventions help a person to formulate their thoughts into an utterance, while other interventions are geared to find an alternative way to natural speech. Which intervention may be effective depends on the needs, the condition, and the prognosis of a person's development.

AAC comes in many shapes and forms. Some people use AAC for just a few utterances, while others use AAC of lectures, and for almost nonstop communication with their partners during every waking moment. Is it even possible to find a commonality between all the forms? We believe that there is: it essentially comes down to the principles of interactive human communication, and the principles of personal message generating.

PRINCIPLE OF INTERACTIVE HUMAN COMMUNICATION

In the summer of 1991, during a 1-month research visit at Purdue University, I was working on explanatory models for AAC. My host Lyle Lloyd convinced me that it would be a mistake to try to grasp AAC as if it is essentially different from typical communication. Both the typical communicator and the AAC user are essentially human minds processing and exchanging information. There is no reason to believe that these processes follow different channels or different laws. This view has helped me in my endeavors to paint a comprehensive picture of AAC. Just as typical communication, it is about externalizing thoughts in a form that can be captured by a communication partner. The forms can vary: they can be spoken or written words, whistles, eye winks, gestures, coughs, facial expressions, text messages, or photographs. Anything works.

This is sometimes called *multimodality*. Very often, people use a combination of forms: most people gesture while they speak, and many throw in an emoticon when they e-mail. In AAC, we often seek for the most efficient and effective combination of communication forms, just as any human communicator does.

Another characteristic of human communication is speed (Reed & Durlach, 1998). Rate of information production needs to be within a range of comfortable information processing to work within live communication setting (i.e., where sender and receiver are present and engaged in interaction). In other words, information exchange should neither go too fast or too slow in order to allow both sender and receiver to process, anticipate, and remember the messages and the flow of conversation. The use of AAC does not always permit to keep conversation within the comfortable range. I believe this is one of the major challenges that we still face in AAC.

PRINCIPLE OF PERSONAL MESSAGE GENERATING

Multimodality is not only a social principle; it is also an *individual* phenomenon. It means that the different modes of communication are part of a person's own repertoire of communication forms. It implies that communication forms are "stored" in the person's mental system in such a way that they can be retrieved and activated for production (or for recognition). Within AAC, "alternative" symbols are often used (e.g., pictures or photographs, graphic symbols). Does the user have a mental representation of these that is similar to words in an internal lexicon?

And how do internalized alternative symbols relate to words? Will they facilitate access to words?

Today's psycholinguistic models attempt to analyze speech and automaticity in communication: how is it possible that most people, when speaking, have little trouble finding the words to say? And how is it that these words seem to fall automatically into syntactic patterns? It is clear that fast internal processes precede the articulation of words. The most used model to describe the microgenesis of speech is Levelt's blueprint of the speaker (1993). This model proposes that the speaker finds the words in an internal lexicon and places them in a syntactic structure or template before actually starting speech. Similarly, AAC users will need to "navigate" their device to find the words or phrase they want to activate. This navigation can simply consist of visually scanning a communication board, but it can also involve different steps through pages on a device to find the symbol that is looked for. Here lies another major challenge for AAC: can AAC compete with the fast lexical access of typical communicators? How can we accelerate access?

THE FUTURE OF AAC

In the past few years (and probably in the near future), applications of AAC have multiplied thanks to more affordable, and faster technology (especially mobile computing and tablet technology). These developments are to be welcomed and encouraged as they make AAC available to more individuals with fewer financial costs. It also "normalizes" AAC more as it blurs the distinction between disabled and nondisabled people since they both use the same type of devices for communication and information storage and processing.

However, these new developments do not fundamentally alter the framework within which AAC is defined: AAC essentially remains an approach of facilitation of information processing and information exchange.

The future of AAC appears to be exciting (Light & McNaughton, 2012). Besides (and partially because of) the increased availability of AAC solutions, a number of other developments are remarkable. Expectations are likely to be higher than ever: if we have more and better tools, we should have better results. Also, the fact that more individuals use AAC solutions, makes it more possible to compare outcomes, which leads to evidence-based practice (Schlosser & Raghavendra, 2004). Finally, I believe that AAC will become more than just an applied discipline. It tells us something about the potential of humans to go beyond standard forms of information exchange in communication. Natural speech will probably remain the standard and the norm of direct human communication. But alternatives to natural speech are just as normal and a testimony of human resilience. The study of AAC use is potentially a very promising data source to understand how people process and structure information that is brought to them through a combination of different modalities.

THE STRUCTURE OF THIS BOOK

This book is organized in 13 chapters, each focusing on a topic that is important to understand AAC. With the exception of Chapters 6 (prelinguistic communication)

and 8 (AAC in individuals with acquired disorders), the information is not organized around a typology or classification of disorders. The structure of the book tries to be consistent with the view that a communication and message generation model should be the basis to understand the possibilities to communicate. In other words, it would be misleading if it were suggested that there are typical or different forms of AAC that apply to individuals with autism spectrum disorders, or other groups. We believe that a carefully analysis of the communication needs as such, together with the possibilities of learning and growth that will determine the nature of the AAC intervention.

Chapter 1 is the introductory chapter in which some of the basic concepts and terminology are explained.

Chapters 2 and 3 present the reader with the issue of access. The chapter employs the blueprint of the speaker, a model proposed by Levelt (1993). This model indicates how speech is the result of a parallel multicomponential process of word and sentence activation. The model is useful to pinpoint where in the process elements are different when nontypical communication (such as manual signs or the activation of a speech-generating device) occurs. Chapter 3 describes where in the process technological prostheses could be inserted to perform parts of the communication process.

Chapter 4 discusses the symbols. Symbols are the units of meaning within a communication system. Spoken or written words are clearly symbols. Specific to AAC, probably the best-known symbols are graphic symbols (pictures, or a graphic representation of an object or idea based), but manual signs, eye-blinking, or other behaviors can also serve as symbols.

Chapter 5 can be seen as an extension of the previous chapter. It focuses on the question how symbols are organized in a coherent way. In spoken and signed languages, words are part of lexicons that are internally organized in such a way that they can easily be accessed. The challenge for AAC is to ensure that the alternative lexicon (graphic symbols, manual signs) is as functional as possible and as easily accessible as words are for a speaker of a spoken language.

Chapter 6 is about prelinguistic development and how AAC techniques can be used to help launch early communicative behaviors, which are typically displayed by children in the first 2 years of life. AAC techniques offer some possibilities to facilitate early communication and the transition from early nonlinguistic to linguistic communication (i.e., use of symbols in a basic grammatical structure).

Chapter 7 addresses questions of language learning and acquisition. In this chapter, we touch on an important discussion: does the use of an "alternative" form of communication lead to a form of structuring information that is different from the structure of spoken language? AAC increases a person's opportunities to express language (and its structures). This allows the environment to respond to the person's utterances and "teach" structures of grammar.

Chapter 8 deals with the issue of needs for alternative forms of communication in individuals with have acquired disorders. This implies that the persons have previously functioned without any need for an alternative mode. How can AAC meet the sudden or gradual changes in language and communication needs?

Chapter 9 discusses the importance and the issues related to literacy development on people who use AAC. Literacy is one of the keys that allows individuals to participate and self-develop. Interest in the importance of literacy for children who use AAC only emerged in the 1990s. Previously, AAC implementation was focused on giving the child the tools for direct face-to-face communication. The chapter analyzes the questions whether young AAC users may be at a disadvantage (or not) in acquiring reading and writing skills.

Chapter 10 addresses the relation between the use of AAC and natural speech. Since I started my professional career in the 1970s, I have been confronted with this interesting and recurring topic. Should we not discourage manual signing, or any use of an alternative form, as it might reduce a person's investment in natural speech. I believe that underlying to this question lays an idea of incompatibility—a strange but widespread opinion in a world with a majority of bilingual people, in a world where everybody uses different ways to express himself or herself. Especially speaking and writing—if I suggested that you should not learn to read and write because it would decrease your motivation to speak, you would think I am crazy. Nevertheless, that is exactly what is often feared. Unfortunately, it has frequently prevented children (and adults) to be offered AAC, while it would most likely have been a help for them.

Chapter 11 focuses on AAC assessment, both as a theoretical and an applied issue. Can AAC performance be measured, and what should be the norms of measurement? Can results of AAC be predicted? Isn't communication, and certainly AAC, idiosyncratic?, Does this mean that communication performance cannot be compared with communication standards? Maybe, what we need in assessment is not so much a measurement of the communication at the time of assessment, but a measurement of the *potential* to use and adapt new forms (alternative and augmentative) of communication.

In Chapter 12, the relation between AAC use and the community is explored. Communication, by definition, is a social activity. Communication is always shared by at least one other person. As a social process, communication is key to participation. Communication (or lack thereof) can reveal much of how people are valued, perceived, and awarded opportunities in communication. Communication also can show equalities and inequalities in how individuals interact. Through the nature of their communication, people who use AAC are not always given and encouraged to participate fully.

In Chapter 13, the focus is on the AAC experience from the perspective of the AAC user. Throughout the chapters, it should have become clear that complex communication needs must have a strong impact on a person's perception of life. Not being an AAC user myself, I felt most hesitant to write about these perspectives as they are, by definition, very personal and can be hardly reported by a third person.

Why are there 13 chapters? After I had been teaching AAC courses for almost 10 years, I was asked to teach an online course. I suddenly realized how much I had relied on the face-to-face contact in the classroom where I can tell students what is important, how I see things, and what I want them to remember. That is when I started to write pages and pages of lecture notes and gave them to the students to study and to solicit their feedback. Thirteen weeks in a semester, 13 chapters in this book. I hope that it offers a framework and can be used as course materials by others.

REFERENCES

Levelt, W. J. M. (1993). *Speaking: From intention to articulation* (1st MIT Pbk. ed.). Cambridge, MA: MIT Press.

Light, J., & McNaughton, D. (2012). The changing face of augmentative and alternative communication: Past, present, and future challenges. *Augmentative and Alternative Communication, 28*(4), 197–204.

McNaughton, D., & Light, J. (2013). The iPad and mobile technology revolution: Benefits and challenges for individuals who require augmentative and alternative communication. *Augmentative and Alternative Communication, 29*(2), 107–116.

Reed, C. M., & Durlach, N. I. (1998). Note on information transfer rates in human communication. *Presence: Teleoperators and Virtual Environments, 7*(5), 509–518.

Schlosser, R. W., & Raghavendra, P. (2004). Evidence-based practice in augmentative and alternative communication. *AAC: Augmentative and Alternative Communication, 20*(1), 1–21.

Acknowledgments

This book is the result of my attempt to find a theoretical, clinical, and educational framework for Augmentative and Alternative Communication in connection with the wider field of education, clinical intervention, and especially communication psychology and psycholinguistics. Over the years mentors, colleagues, students, lab members, and friends have helped me in trying to find a framework to understand AAC. I am grateful to all of them! I especially want to thank Lyle Lloyd, who ignited my interest in the explanatory models back in the 1990s.

I thank the AAC users whom I have met in committees and at conferences. Thanks are especially due to those who became friends. They made AAC more personal to me and are always living demonstrations of how vital communication is.

The book has grown out of my lectures in AAC at the University of Virginia, James Madison University, and Longwood University, as well as from presentations and talks I have given at several conferences. I have learned a tremendous amount from the interactions with my students, their feedback, and their insistence on connecting theory with clinical, educational, and social applications. I appreciate their willingness to accept that I had more hypotheses than definite certainties to offer.

I thank my editors at Plural, especially Milgem and Valerie, for their help, their patience, encouragements, and professionalism. Chelsea Bachman, Aja Walker, and Taylor Levine have read and edited earlier versions of the chapters, and helped with the bibliographic references. My gratitude goes also to my son-artist Joris Loncke for his many illustrations for this book and for other projects in the past and hopefully in the future.

And most of all, very special thanks go to you, Lee, for your gentle encouragement, your patience, and, always, your understanding and love.

—Filip Loncke, PhD

CHAPTER 1

AAC: A General Introduction

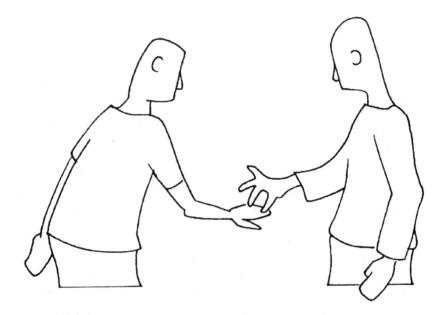

The term *Augmentative and Alternative Communication* (AAC) refers to the methods, tools, and theories of the use of nonstandard linguistic and nonlinguistic forms of communication by and with individuals without or with limited functional speech (Figure 1–1).

Methods include: (1) the use of nonstandard modalities (e.g., the use of manual signs or the use of a speech-generating communication device); (2) the "materialization" of the communication act (e.g., picture or token exchange between sender and receiver to make the communication "tangible"), and (3) the modification of any parameter in the communication (e.g., bringing nonverbal communication forms more to the foreground in communication; e.g., the use of eye-gaze).

The *tools* are generally what makes AAC stand out as specific way of intervention or communicating. AAC tools include a variety of materials and devices varying from nontech, such as communication symbol cards and a communication vest, to low-tech means such as one-message switches, to high-tech computer-based communication devices. The tools of AAC also include any repertoire of communication *forms* such as manual signs, eye signaling codes, and basic nonlinguistic vocalizations.

Theories try to explain the differences and similarities between the use of AAC and typical forms communication.

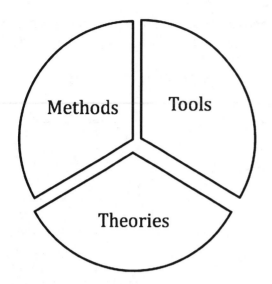

Figure 1–1. AAC methods, tools, and theories.

For example, theories will attempt to explain how the different modalities work together in the mind of the AAC user. This includes the discussion about the compatibility of manual sign and speech (are they mutually reinforcing or are they competitors?)—a controversy among educators that goes back more than two centuries. Theories also include the study of the impact on language acquisition by AAC users, the social impact for the AAC user, educational aspects such as AAC and literacy, AAC in the classroom, and the social perception and attitudes of communication partners. Theories should account for differences and similarities among groups of AAC users: children (who are to acquire language), adults, and individuals with neurogenic communication disorders (who may have lost linguistic or communicative functions).

In short, theories provide a framework that helps us to explain how AAC works. Theories are important, as they help predict and explain progress, as well as failure. Evidence and data result-

ing from observation can corroborate or weaken theories. For example, in the past, the use of alternative modes of communication was frequently considered to interfere negatively with the development of speech articulation skills. Underlying this opinion was the hypothesis that modalities are mutually exclusive and have a degree of incompatibility. However, observations and analysis of systematic studies of users of AAC now call for a revision of such theoretical assumptions: modalities appear to operate in a mutually reinforcing way (Millar, Light, & Schlosser, 2006).

Although the term AAC was not coined and used until the early 1980s, the concept of using nonstandard communication forms to help individuals without or with limited speech has been around for centuries. Although "AAC" is usually not the term used for the most obvious and well-known solution for individuals with severe hearing impairment, the use of manual signing (sign languages such as American Sign Language [ASL]) in educational programs for deaf children is nevertheless based on the same principle as AAC: Identify and use the most accessible modality (visual-gestural) to enable cognitive, social, linguistic, and academic development. The use of this principle goes back at least 250 years.

STANDARD AND NONSTANDARD FORMS OF COMMUNICATION

Standard linguistic forms of communication are speech/listening and writing/reading. We call them standard forms because they appear to be the most effective linguistic forms for typical language users.

Nonstandard forms of communication include gestures, vocalizations, body positions and body orientation, the use of graphic symbols, and eye gazing.

In the past two decades, electronic forms of communication have entered the realm of typical communication including e-mailing (computer-to-computer communication), and, increasingly, mobile computing. These developments continue to have an enormous impact on AAC as they have helped to widen the selection of possibilities for individuals who need AAC. For example, the advent of tablet computing is considered by many to have dramatically changed the AAC world in terms of availability, cost structure, client-clinician relationship, and acceptability. New developments have also improved the quality of AAC technology. For instance, the improvement of intelligibility of digitized AAC speech is largely the result of mainstream research and development.

AAC is meant for *individuals without speech or with limited functional speech.* Although this is seldom explicitly described or mentioned, its traditional users —understand the term "traditional" in the meaning "most often thought of"— are persons whose language and communication are not expected to progress significantly to enable them to fully realize their communicative, linguistic, and social potential. In the 1970s, during the earliest stages of AAC history, nonspeaking children and adults with cerebral palsy, whose speech limitations are clearly not due to linguistic, cognitive, or social impairments, were often the first to adopt AAC.

EARLY ASSUMPTIONS

This early view on the target user of AAC reveals three assumptions, all of which have rightly been refuted in the past three decades, extending AAC in its use and applications.

1. Early assumption #1. The success of AAC solutions depends on the cognitive and linguistic skills as well as the motivation of the AAC user. Although this is certainly true, it tends to underestimate the crucial role that is played by the communication partners. One cannot play tennis without a partner. If the communication partner has low expectations, does not respond, or does not provide communication opportunities, the AAC user's development will suffer. In other words, we cannot put all the burden of success on the shoulders of the user. The communication partners and the environment will bear a very important responsibility.

2. Early assumption #2. AAC needs not to be considered until more traditional speech and language intervention methods have failed. This "last resort" approach has often wasted important developmental potential in AAC users. Sometimes, practitioners would put off the introduction of AAC because they feared that it would make young AAC users digress from normal development. An underlying fear was that there would be an incompatibility between natural speech and alternative forms of communication. Today, there is growing evidence that: (1) there is no incompatibility between modalities and that (2) the use of a highly accessible modality reinforces early development. One striking development is that parents of typically developing children use Baby Signs to improve early communication and to accelerate

the transition from prelinguistic to linguistic communication (Goodwyn, Acredolo, & Brown, 2000). The underlying vision has shifted. Initially, it was feared that alternative forms of communication would get in the way of normal speech development. This general conviction has been contested for a simple reason: More accessible modalities have the potential to provide the child with experience in social exchanges (dialogues), naming, and self-expression. These experiences facilitate the transition to language. Applied to AAC, the early introduction of accessible communication is beneficial for social, linguistic, and cognitive development.

3. Early assumption #3. AAC was originally considered to be just about communication. AAC was considered to be something to remove a barrier, after which the actual intervention (linguistic, cognitive, social) could start. Today, AAC is more and more considered to be an integral part of the intervention itself. For example, graphic symbols are now used in a wide range of didactic and educational tools, including schedules (Figure 1–2), calendars, and planning tools.

TERMINOLOGY

To understand AAC, it may be useful to focus on a few key terms:

- *Aided communication:* Refers to the use of aids external to the communicator's body, for example: symbol cards, a notebook, a speech-generating communication device.
- *Unaided communication:* Refers to communication that is entirely established without external aids such as natural speech, sign language, gesturing.

Does the distinction between aided and unaided communication matter? Some practitioners have argued that it does. The fact that unaided communication is at all times available to the person,

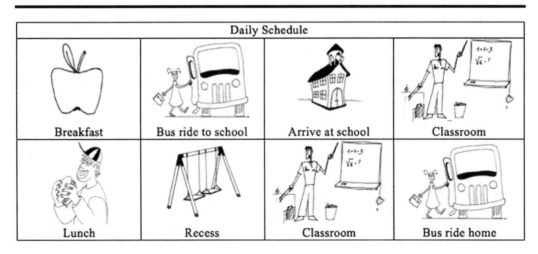

Figure 1–2. A communication board as a schedule.

is an important factor. It is suspected that unaided communication might be more natural and easier for maintaining eye-to-eye communication. However, with miniaturization of devices, it is not clear if this difference still has the same importance as it once had (see Chapter 3).

The following terms have been suggested and used to describe the person who uses AAC: *AAC user*, *consumer*, and *person who uses AAC*. More recently, the term person with *complex communication needs* (CCN) has been suggested and is increasingly used in the literature. The question is whether this term accurately describes "the" AAC user. For example, Lloyd (personal communication, 2012) points out that a person who has severe speech fluency problems could be characterized as having complex communication needs even though one would generally not think that this person would need AAC. More recently, the obvious term "People who use Augmentative and Alternative Communication" has been used (e.g., at the 2012 convention of the International Society for Augmentative and Alternative Communication). In this book, we use the more neutral terms "people who use AAC," or "AAC user."

Other terms that are relevant to understand AAC include: *Communication*, *Speech*, and *Language*. *Communication* is the term used to indicate the exchange of information between at least two partners. AAC uses both linguistic and nonlinguistic means of communication. Communication can be linguistic (using language) or nonlinguistic (using all other forms of behaviors). *Language* refers to a socially shared code that is a specific rule-governed system consisting of phonology, a lexicon, morphology, and syntax. Many psycholinguists believe that language is a uniquely human system that only humans possess. *Speech* is one modality to express language. Speech is the result of encoding phonological sequences into articulatory gestures. It can be considered to be the preferred way of language output because it is rapid and effective, and because it is naturally embedded in face-to-face interaction. Speech is also relatively effortless—at least for a majority of language users. However, in cases where speech is not an obvious and easy output of language, there are alternatives: the use of manual signing, the use of picture communication, the use of speech generating devices—each of these have the potential to carry linguistic information. In fact, every literate language speaker uses alternatives for natural speech all the time such as writing letters, notes, e-mails, and by text messaging.

Another—sometimes confusing—term is *symbol*. In cognitive psychology, a symbol is most often defined as something that refers to or represents an object, a person, or an idea. A symbol is essentially a referential tool. The symbolic value is the result of a connection that someone makes with a referent. Strictly speaking, a symbol is something that can only exist in your head. For example, a picture of a banana can be a symbol for you—because you recognize the picture and make the connection with things that you have encountered in the world, that is, bananas. However, if a person lacks the recognition skills that are required to "decode" the picture—there is research exploring when in the course of the first months and years a typical person is able to recognize a picture (DeLoache, 2011)—then the picture is meaningless. In AAC, the term "symbol" or "graphic symbol" is used for pictures or graphic representations. It is important to keep in mind that these symbols may not have any symbolic value at all for individuals functioning at a presymbolic level. In some cases, neurological damage can also cause impairment of symbolic functions, sometimes called asymbolia.

That being said, within AAC, a distinction is sometimes made between a *symbol set* and a *symbol system*. A symbol set is a collection of graphic symbols that do not have any internal principles regarding symbol formation. For example, a speech-language pathologist who would make her own collection of symbols by making drawings, taking photographs, and by cutting pictures from magazines and children's books has built a symbol set. A *symbol system*, on the other hand, will use rules to build the pictures. For example, in the *Bliss words* system (see Chapter 4), a man is a simple intuitive "stick figure" with a little circle as head, and straight lines for the body and the legs. A woman is exactly the same figure with only a triangle over the legs (representing a skirt). Both graphic symbols have a lot in common—not only conceptually but also formationally, that is, in the way the graphic symbol is built. The two symbols are minimal pairs, contrasting through one characteristic.

AAC is often thought of as *nonverbal communication*. The terms verbal and nonverbal are somewhat ambiguous. The Latin word *Verbum* means "word." However, the term verbal is used with varying meanings, such as "with words," "with spoken words," "with language," and "academically" (for example, as in the Wechsler verbal intelligence scales; Baker, 1980). Therefore, it is not clear if the sign languages of deaf communication should be considered to be "verbal" or not. Sign languages are linguistic systems, but they do not use "words" in the narrow sense.

With the ambiguity surrounding nonverbal communication, the term should not be used to refer to AAC to avoid misunderstandings and misinterpretations.

The terms *vocal* and *nonvocal* are more specific as they refer to the presence or absence of natural speech. They indicate whether communication is produced with the human voice. The distinction *linguistic–nonlinguistic* is also useful as it refers to whether linguistic principles are underlying the communication. An internal linguistic "engine" most likely drives the utterances of users of sign language and natural speakers. On the other hand, a single gesture, pointing, and the use of simple picture communication exchange may or may not be based on a person's linguistic system. If a person uses a few words, a few gestures, or points to a few pictures, it may not be clear whether this is the mere result of association between a behavior and a result, or whether the person uses internalized language-like rules (e.g., subject-verb structures).

LEARNABILITY OF SYMBOLS

One of the reasons why graphic symbols and manual signs are often used in AAC is the presumed easy learnability. While most spoken words have a purely arbitrary and conventional relationship with their referent, manual signs and graphic symbols can be more "iconic." *Iconicity* means that the symbol has image-value. *Transparency* implies that you can "look through" the symbol and immediately extract its meaning. Examples of transparency are: a picture of a house (meaning: house, obviously!) and the manual sign for drink (pretending you are drinking from a cup—meaning: drink!). A symbol is said to be *translucent* when the relationship with the meaning only becomes obvious after one reveals it. For example, the ASL sign for YEAR is produced by holding one fist steady while the other fist makes a rotation around it (Figure 1–3). When explained that this symbolizes the earth's rotation around the sun, the sign acquires iconic value for many learners and users.

Manual signs and sign language are specific uses of *gestures*. What are *gestures*? Are they different from manual signs? *Gesture* is a general term for movements that are made with hands and arms, often accompanied with facial expressions. Gestures may look like manual signs, but they do not need to have a specific linguistic meaning. In the past three decades, psychologists have become increasingly fascinated by the gesture phenomenon.

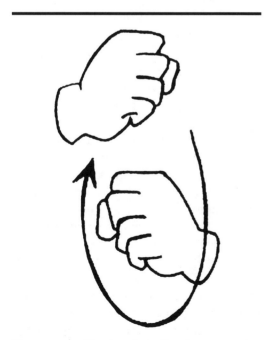

Figure 1–3. The American Sign Language sign YEAR.

Everybody uses gestures, as they often accompany natural speech. Gestures can carry a specific meaning, but this is not always the case. Sometimes information carried and conveyed by gestures is redundant with the information of the spoken message, and sometimes it is complementary. Gestures appear to be more intuitive than speech—speakers are often not even aware that they are gesturing. McNeill (1992) argues that gestures offer a window to the mind. Gesture and speech are used all the time together. The natural combination and concurrence of gesture and speech illustrates the human tendency for synchronous multimodal expression and communication. Gestures also become more salient when it is needed to make the communication more effective. For example, when a person gives directions to a location, he or she needs to provide "spatial information." This will likely cause a person to use more gestures—even if one is talking on the phone (where the communication partner can clearly not benefit from it).

While many gestures are idiosyncratic or have no meaning at all (e.g., the "beats"—movements of speakers when emphasizing a point they want to make), some gestures reflect something that the speaker wants to convey (e.g., iconic gestures for "ball," or metaphoric gestures for "a big idea"). Each culture contains a limited number of gestures with a well-defined meaning. These gestures, or *emblems*, function as single words with a specific meaning, such as "excellent" (thumbs up), "disgust" (finger pointing into mouth), and other well-known obscene gestures.

In some cases of natural and typical communication, gestures replace speech entirely. This natural tendency is elevated to a principle of practice in AAC. In many applications, AAC uses a nonspeech modality (gesture, manual sign, a picture) along with speech. In other words, AAC uses a natural phenomenon and reinforces it in an organized and systematic way.

A *manual sign* is a gesture that has become conventionalized (when several users agree on the meaning), and that has become an integrated part of the lexicon of a visual-gestural language, that is, a sign language. ASL, along with many other sign languages that have emerged in deaf communities in the world, is one example of a full-fledged language in the visual-gestural modality. Special educators have sometimes promoted the use of *sign systems*, where signs are used and organized in the structure of the spoken language (e.g., *Signed English*). The purpose of these systems has always been "pedagogical": It would supposedly allow the use of *simultaneous communication* (speaking and signing at the same time) and would make the structure of the spoken language more visible. The results and the validity of this rationale have long been a matter of debate within the world of deaf education.

The practice of *simultaneous communication* has been largely adopted within AAC. The underlying assumption is that individuals tend to function in a *multimodal* way. *Multimodality* (Loncke, Campbell, England, & Haley, 2006) refers to the fact that more than one channel is used for communication (gesture, speech, picture, a communication device). Multimodality also refers to the hypothesis that language users have multiple internal symbolic representations inside their heads, and that these representations are internally organized in a network. For example, speaking a word and pointing to a picture would

strengthen an internal link—speech would then potentially benefit from the use of the other modality. This view is opposed to the *incompatibility hypothesis*, which states that the different modalities are in competition with one another, and that learning one modality will suppress the acquisition of the other modality. The incompatibility belief has been dominant for decades, resulting in advice at times given to parents to not use manual signs—as it was supposed to be detrimental to the acquisition of speech. At present, most evidence points in the direction of compatibility between modalities (the relation and the dynamics between the modalities is, however, probably much more complex than stated here). AAC practitioners will certainly be questioned by parents and relatives of their clients—but also sometimes by their own peers—about the "risks for natural speech" of the use of alternatives for speech.

Total communication is a somewhat older term used to indicate the educational and clinical philosophy of maximally exploiting the possibilities of speech with the most workable and effective combination and configuration of other modalities.

For many observers, AAC is equated with the use of electronic communication devices. Although assistive communication technology is certainly an important and growing aspect of AAC, the field focuses in the first place on how and when to use methods and materials that supplement or substitute for speech. Electronic devices are only part of the story. The term presently used for these devices—and accepted (e.g., for insurance funding)—is *speech-generating communication device* (SGD). Older terms are VOCA (*voice-output communication aid*) and, simply, speech-device. Sometimes a distinction is made between a *dedicated communication device* and a *nondedicated communication device*. A dedicated device is uniquely built and used as a communication tool, whereas a nondedicated communication device can have other applications. Most commonly, nondedicated communication devices use a laptop computer or mobile computing tablet platform, which potentially allows the user to use other computer applications than just the communication software.

has been wrapped (encoded) by the sender—and that the receiver thus gets to the original idea of the sender. This is arguably not the case for any communication (see e.g., Pinker, 2007), and it is most likely not what happens in AAC (where the encoder might be limited by the choices offered by a device). Nevertheless, the sender-message-receiver model is adequate, as it allows us to describe a number of characteristics of AAC. In the following section, this framework is used to describe some of the application areas of AAC.

A MODEL FOR AAC COMMUNICATION

In 1990, Lloyd, Quist, and Windsor (1990) proposed a model to describe AAC. Rather than characterizing AAC as a phenomenon that cannot be grasped by the traditional communication models, they argued that the essence of AAC can be described by the "sender-message-receiver" model (Figure 1–4). Admittedly, the model does have its limitations: for example, it is naïve to suppose that any communication consists of a process where the receiver "unwraps" (decodes) the message as if it was a package that

AAC AS SENDER SUPPORT

Most of the applications of AAC are intended to help people express what they want to say (i.e., they provide sender support). That can happen at several levels in the process of generating a message. In typical speech communication, a speaker goes through several operations toward the production of a message, which usually include: (1) having an intention (I want to say something), (2) finding a (syntactic) structure (Do I want a statement, a question, a command?), (3) finding the words for what I want to say in the

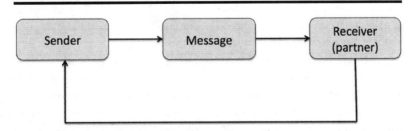

Figure 1–4. The Sender–Message–Receiver model.

internal lexicon, (4) putting the words in order and marking them morphologically (plurals, word endings), (5) identifying the phonological structure and forming a phonetic plan, and then—finally—(6) activating the speech articulators based on the phonetic plan.

Individuals with AAC needs may have problems in message generating at one or more of the above successive steps and levels. It may simply be that the process—which normally is a matter of microseconds—goes too fast, and that a visual help is needed to keep them focused on the process.

One application of AAC is to help the person establish *intentionality* (i.e., the understanding that specific behaviors can have a meaning and can be consequential). This is a domain where specialists in prelinguistic communication, autism, and severe developmental disabilities have worked to establish techniques to teach individuals to mentally make the connection between behavior and consequence: (between "I do something" and "They will do something in response"). This is a form of cause-effect understanding. Many of the basic AAC techniques and tools (e.g., switches) are used to strengthen and practice this understanding and behavior.

Another example of sender-support is vocabulary, which is often made accessible by the use of communication boards or displays (a real board or a computer/tablet screen) that have some representation of a possible lexicon. Researchers have been debating for many years what exactly should go on these boards. There are several issues (all unresolved) that relate to this question. Generally, there is consensus that the *visualization* of the lexicon (the graphic symbols) is useful—presumably as it can serve as an external representation and memory aid of the lexicon. There is, however, quite some discussion about *extent and limitation*—how many graphic symbols can one manage? When are there too many and when is it not enough? An important consideration is that typical children at the age of five already know and use thousands of words. If we don't represent all of these words, are we shortchanging a child? If so, how do we make all of the vocabulary accessible? Organizationally and logistically, it may simply not be doable to give a child a picture dictionary of thousands of entries—how would they manage this? Will it simply discourage communication (help! how do you want me to find the words I am supposed to say!)? The problem is that the typical (internalized) mental lexicon is very flexible and well organized, which makes quick and easy access the rule and not the exception. Communication devices, even computerized pages with displays, do not offer an equal alternative. Often, communication devices contain graphic symbols that are represented and organized in screens (computer pages) where the user needs to learn and remember the *navigation* principles to identify the symbols. Not only is this taxing the memory, but it is most of all a challenge to the need for rapid communication.

LESS IS MORE?

Some AAC approaches imply that we should adopt a *less-is-more* philosophy. Instead of overwhelming the user with many graphic symbols, we should limit the number of symbols to a *core vocabulary*. A core vocabulary should contain words and phrases that are useful to get people through their daily life and activities. Instead of teaching and learning many words, the user will have to learn strategies to say many things with a limited number of words.

Another alternative has also been applied. Instead of having to choose between multitudes of symbols that are unmanageable or a limited number that will cause frustration, some educators suggest that the solution lies in the combinatoriality principle: to create words and phrases by combining elements of the selection set. One clear example is the use of the alphabetic principle. Literate AAC users often employ letter boards or devices, which have a typical computer keyboard. By pointing to the letters of the alphabet, the user is able to form words. When you type the message on a device, it appears on a screen and it can be activated into speech output. This is one reason why literacy needs to be a prime objective in intervention and education of AAC users. Literacy will empower and increase the possibilities for expression. However, some AAC users may not be able to become literate. Bruce Baker (2012), a linguist, developed an icon-based combinatorial system, called Minspeak. Although the system was originally intended for literate users for rate enhancement, it can be a significant help for nonreading people. Minspeak, installed on communication devices from Prentke Romich Company, is a system that allows users to combine a limited number of graphic symbols in order to generate a range of meanings. The user does not have to remember the location of hundreds of graphic symbols. Instead, the user simply needs to know the combination code to create the words or phrases (see Chapter 2).

Finally, a number of AAC studies have focused on the *representation* issue of graphic symbols. When are graphic symbols most effective and most learnable? Often the answer has been related to the iconicity issue. The stronger and easier the relation is between the symbol and the meaning, the more likely that it will be used and remembered. However, it is hard to find graphic symbols that are unambiguous. Moreover, iconicity is almost impossible to achieve for verbs. How do you represent "jump" (or any movement verb, for that matter)? Other aspects of graphic symbols that have been researched are the effect of color, size, and the difference between photographs and drawings.

There have been similar discussions concerning the lexicon of manual signs: should we offer a limited lexicon (a number that is often suggested is 500 signs) and teach the users ways to express as much as possible with this basic lexicon, or should we offer an unlimited number of signs—according to the person's learning potential?

ALTERNATIVE ACCESS

An essential feature of AAC systems is that it offers an expressive mode that may be accessible for a user with limitations. For example, we need a solution for the fact that many AAC users have trouble with the motor act of speaking. Therefore, we need alternative access, which is often done by offering the person to access and build messages through pointing or through touching (of a screen). Pointing does not need to be finger pointing. It can be eye-gaze pointing too. In the nontech form, a communication partner observes in which direction the person is looking and determines what the person tries to say. This is called *partner-assisted communication* because the communication partner takes over some of the burden of the message construction. Strategies can be developed and agreed upon; for example, if provided with a roster of symbols (e.g., five rows of five symbols), the first step might be to determine the row where the targeted symbol is, followed by the second step (i.e., if one wants the first, the second, the third, . . . in the row). Advanced electronic devices are now commonly equipped with eye gaze sensors that can be activated to follow the person's gaze and to activate a symbol if the person's eyes dwell for one or two seconds on a location, if a person blinks, or another eye behavior.

In short, AAC may attempt to reduce the motor requirements for expressing a message by looking for alternatives. This is also part of the rationale why manual signs are often used with and by nonspeaking individuals with autism and developmental disabilities. Because manual signs are produced with muscle groups that are situated more on the periphery of the body (control of the arms, the fingers, the shoulders), they are presumably somewhat easier to produce than natural speech—which is considered one of the most complex and highly coordinated motor activities. This explains why typically developing children can learn a few manual signs prior to being able to speak their first words, an observation that has been put into practice by many parents of normal children who have adopted baby signs (Goodwyn et al., 2000).

Adapting Manual Signs

The signs of sign languages, such as ASL, may not always be that easy to execute by individuals with development limitations. Many of the signs of ASL and other sign languages require coordination of two moving hands as well as the ability to assume different hand configurations (e.g., the so called G-hand, where index finger and thumb are extended). Therefore, educators have proposed the use of somewhat modified manual signs that would accommodate the need for motor simplicity by individuals with developmental limitations. One example is the Simplified Sign System, developed at the University of Virginia by John Bonvillian and his associates (Bonvillian et al., 2009). Bonvillian looked up signs from 41 different sign languages around the world to pick those signs that appeared to be the easiest to execute. Then, he tested the signs with hundreds of undergraduate students to determine which ones were easiest to make and which ones were easiest to remember. This approach led to a lexicon of about 1,000 manual signs, which are to be used in the communication by and with individuals who have little or no functional natural speech.

AAC AS SUPPORT OF SIGNAL TRANSMISSION

A crucial aspect of communication is the transmission of the message from the sender to the receiver. Some AAC interventions are focused on facilitating this part of the process. Many are plain common sense. For example, you may simply want to make the signal more distinguishable by speaking more slowly or by sound amplification. Speaking more slowly allows the receiver more time to decide what the signal is. In typical speech, speakers can easily say 200 or more words a minute. Listeners generally have no trouble in deciding what they are hearing. However, if English is not your native language, you might appreciate it if speakers slow down a little bit (this is true for any foreign language you are learning—remember your high school experience/trauma with language classes). Also, speaking more loudly, repetition, and other forms of reinforcement help to bring the spoken signal to the foreground, facilitating comprehension of what the signal is.

One well-known technique within AAC is the *materialized exchange of messages* through message cards (e.g., PECS, the Picture Exchange Communication System; Bondy & Frost, 1994). The technique materializes the act of exchanging a message in communication by literally handing it over from sender to receiver (remember that the exchange of most messages in communication is an invisible process—except for traditional snail mail, you cannot see the message move from sender to receiver). Techniques such as the *materialized exchange of messages* supposedly help individuals with cognitive-social limitations to grasp the concept of what communication is and how they can play an active role in it.

Multimodality

Lastly, the already mentioned multimodality is one of the strong features of AAC. Although it can be argued that typical communication is already multimodal (after all, speakers assume body positions, gesture, smile, point, draw, and so on while they are addressing their listeners), in AAC one systematically attempts to identify which modalities to use in which configuration.

AAC AS SUPPORT OF RECEIVER

Many of the same measures to facilitate the sender and the signal transmission also apply to the receiver. The receiver's task is to: (1) pay attention to the signals, (2) decode them, and (3) make sense of them. Again, receivers will find themselves in a more comfortable position if the signal is clear (in the foreground) and produced at a decodable speed (not too fast). Graphic symbols have the advantage that they are static: they do not fluctuate or vary in how they are performed, which makes identification easier. Also, it has been argued that the use of a limited lexicon has the advantage that it will be easier to identify which symbols are presented.

BEYOND THE COMMUNICATOR— PARTNER INTERACTION

Thus far, we have talked about AAC as a phenomenon that occurs in the limited realm of people with little or no functional natural speech and their communication partners. While this is an essential part of AAC, it is not complete picture.

Let's raise two questions: (1) why is it that AAC users often abandon their devices? And (2) why is it that AAC users have trouble finding employment? These observations, while unfortunate, are very real and cannot be explained within the sender-message-receiver model. We need to look at it from other, broader perspectives.

AAC abandonment—several reasons have been suggested and probably all of them are true. One reason is simply that effective communication in a social context requires speed of processing and that the AAC solutions often times just fall short of that. Both the AAC users and the listeners may find it not worth the effort to work so hard on constructing a message. Why do nondisabled people talk so much (sometimes thousands of words a day)? Because it is easy (not much effort) and because you get so much out of it (social recognition, information exchange, boss other people around, food, and so on). The balance starts to shift when it becomes more laborious and more painful. Is it really so important for me to crack this joke if I have to work on it for five minutes? Another cause of AAC abandonment might be that AAC forces people (especially the communication partners) out of their habits.

AAC and employment—Why are individuals who are users of AAC often unemployed? There are success stories of AAC users who are employed, self-employed, or have leadership positions. Unfortunately, there is a much greater number of individuals who don't get a paid position. For more than 10 years now, the organization SHOUT has organized the biennial Pittsburgh Employment Conference that is exclusively focused on issues of work for and by AAC users. The fact that such a conference is needed is an illustration and a reminder that AAC use is often perceived as standing in the way of successful economic participation and integration.

Bronfenbrenner's Ecological Model

One way to look at AAC from a wider angle is by adopting Bronfenbrenner's (2006) ecological model. It describes an individual in a central position around which different, wider circles of influence exist (Figure 1–5).

In the center of this model, the individual is located in the *microlevel*. This is the level of the person himself or herself and the person's own characteristics —where we tend to look and identify the features that matter. Traditionally, professionals focus on the microlevel to diagnose and predict a person's success with AAC. Professionals look at a person's linguistic, cognitive, perceptual, motor, and social skills—this assessment will help decide which kinds of assistance will be needed by the person. Light (1989) identified four types of competencies that will matter for an AAC user. These are *linguistic competence* (the ability to identify words and symbols, assemble words into sentences, and so on—things that one measures with language tests), *operational competence* (referring to the ability to use the tools to communicate—that is, does one have the skills to touch buttons to use the device, and so on), *social competence* (communication requires an understanding of the dynamics of social interaction), and *strategic competence* (knowing how to get things done with the AAC system—one could also call this pragmatic competence).

Can we predict a person's AAC success or failure with this information? Probably not (or at least not entirely). Much will depend on how the person's environment will respond to the person using a different way of communication. This brings us to the *mesolevel*—the level of the person in interaction with his or her communication partners in the daily environment. How acceptable is the new communication method for the people in the AAC user's environment? Do they feel comfortable about it, or is there some degree of embarrassment? Or could it be that the communication partners have the best intentions

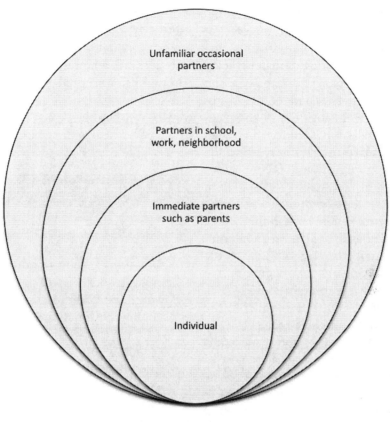

Figure 1–5. Bronfenbrenner's ecological model applied to AAC.

but simply cannot change their habits of years of ignoring an AAC user (who did not speak). The communication partners have to change their perception of the AAC user from seeing him or her as a nonspeaker to someone who can and will speak. Expectations need to change, expectations matter.

The *exolevel* is the wider context in which a person functions. Things that are important at this level are: (1) the degree of (in-)dependence of the person—the more independent one lives, the more one is forced to communicate to get one's needs met, the (2) time schedule in which a person functions (how many opportu-

nities for communication are there?), and (3) economic affordability of health care and AAC provisions.

Finally, at the *macrolevel*, we find factors such as the social perception of an individual who uses an alternative form of communication (how acceptable is it to be different?), the degree to which social inclusion or exclusion of individuals with a disability exists, employment opportunities, market-mechanisms, and the recognition of rights of individuals with a disability. Note that individuals with limited or no functional speech are among the most vulnerable for a wide variety of abuses (financial, social, sexual, physical, and psychological abuse). The implementation of AAC should not only be targeted at giving a person a voice, but also at giving a person the tools to distinguish between appropriate and inappropriate behavior, and to respond (protest and report) appropriately. The American Speech-Language-Hearing Association (ASHA) has been instrumental in drawing attention to the rights to communication by all individuals with AAC needs (ASHA National Joint Committee for the Communication Needs of Persons with Severe Disabilities, 1992). This right is now recognized at an international worldwide level, promoted by the International Society for Augmentative and Alternative Communication (ISAAC), which has successfully brought it to the attention of the United Nations.

To sum up, AAC is about methods, tools, and theories surrounding the use of nonstandard linguistic and nonlinguistic forms of communication by and with individuals without or with limited functional speech. AAC offers a wealth of possibilities for individuals who otherwise might have limitations in communication and in their self-realization. AAC is a fairly new branch within speech-language pathology, special education, and rehabilitation sciences. It is often insufficiently understood, even by practitioners. Romski and Sevcik (2005) have listed a number of myths about AAC, which are important to be aware of. These myths include the assumption that one should not start with AAC intervention until all other options have been exhausted. Or, the fear that natural speech will be impeded once alternative modalities are used. These and other myths are discussed in later chapters of this volume.

Finally, besides the clinical and educational possibilities of AAC, it also provides us with an exciting intellectual and scientific perspective. AAC explores the flexibility and the resilience that humans have to organize and structure their communication. When the standard forms of communication are not available, humans can elevate other modalities and reconfigure them to establish valuable communication and to realize their human potential.

POINTS TO REMEMBER

■ AAC is the term used for the methods, the tools, and the theories of the use of nonstandard linguistic and nonlinguistic forms of communication by and with individuals without or with limited functional speech.

■ AAC taps into a person's ability to combine multiple modalities of expression to form a communication message.

■ AAC does not impede the development of natural speech.

■ AAC is more likely to be effective if it is introduced in an early stage of development or after a communication disability has been detected.

■ The sender-message-receiver model is an adequate framework to comprehend AAC as interventions or modifications at the level of the sender, the message transmission, or the sender.

REFERENCES

ASHA National Joint Committee for the Communication Needs of Persons with Severe Disabilities. (1992). *Communication bill of rights.* Retrieved from http://www.asha.org/NJC/bill_of_rights.htm

Baker, B. (2012). *How minspeak allows for independent communication by giving anyone access to core vocabulary.* Message posted to http://www.minspeak.com/CoreVocabulary.php

Baker, C. (1980). On the terms verbal and nonverbal. In I. Ahlgren & B. Bergman (Eds.), *Papers from the First International Symposium on Sign Language Research.* Stockholm: Swedish National Association of the Deaf.

Bondy, A. S., & Frost, L. A. (1994). The picture exchange communication system. *Focus on Autistic Behavior, 9*(3), 1–19.

Bonvillian, J. D., Dooley, T., Emmons, H., Jack, A., Kissane, N., & Loncke, F. (2009). The development of a simplified manual sign communication system for special populations. *2008 Clinical AAC Research Conference.* Charlottesville, Virginia.

Bronfenbrenner, U. (2006). The bioecological model of human development. In *Handbook of child psychology* (pp. 793–828). Hoboken, NJ: Wiley [Imprint].

DeLoache, J. S. (2011). Early development of the understanding and use of symbolic artifacts. *The Wiley-Blackwell handbook of childhood cognitive development* (2nd ed., pp. 312–336). New York, NY: Wiley-Blackwell.

Goodwyn, S. W., Acredolo, L. P., & Brown, C. A. (2000). Impact of symbolic gesturing on early language development. *Journal of Nonverbal Behavior, 24*(2), 81–103.

Light, J. (1989). Toward a definition of communicative competence for individuals using augmentative and alternative communication systems. *Augmentative and Alternative Communication, 5,* 137–144.

Lloyd, L. (2012). *About the term complex communication needs (CCN).* Personal communication.

Lloyd, L. L., Quist, R. W., & Windsor, J. (1990). A proposed augmentative and alternative communication model. *Augmentative and Alternative Communication, 6*(3), 172.

Loncke, F. T., Campbell, J., England, A. M., & Haley, T. (2006). Multimodality: A basis for augmentative and alternative communication—Psycholinguistic, cognitive, and clinical/educational aspects. *Disability and Rehabilitation, 28*(3), 169–174.

McNeill, D. (1992). *Hand and mind: What gestures reveal about thought.* Chicago, IL: University of Chicago Press.

Millar, D. C., Light, J. C., & Schlosser, R. W. (2006). The impact of augmentative and alternative communication intervention on the speech production of individuals with developmental disabilities: A research review. *Journal of Speech, Language, and Hearing Research, 49*(2), 248–264.

Pinker, S. (2007). *The stuff of thought. Language as a window into human nature.* New York, NY: Viking.

Romski, M., & Sevcik, R. A. (2005). Augmentative communication and early intervention: Myths and realities. *Infants & Young Children, 18*(3), 174–185.

CHAPTER 2

Access and Message Management

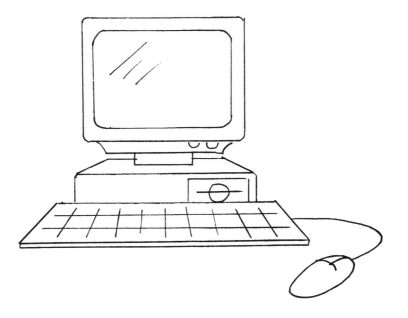

The terms "augmentative" and "alternative" imply that the person, who uses AAC, does something that is different from typical communication. Most of the time, this is easy to *observe*: the person uses a communication device, produces manual signs, points to a graphic symbol, and so on. This is an important part of AAC: the *behavior* that is displayed to communicate may be different from what you see in typical communication. This is one aspect that is discussed in this chapter on access. It is related to *physical access*.

But there is more: how much of the processes that underlie and direct this behavior is different? Is the planning, timing, and coordination of the message formulation similar or different from natural spoken communication? This is *mental access*. In this chapter, we argue that AAC cannot be fully understood if we do not also pay attention to mental processes like word (or symbol) retrieval, combination of symbols, and short-term memory management.

TYPICAL PROCESSES INVOLVED IN THE MICROGENESIS OF SPEECH

For the casual observer, the speed at which typical speech is produced makes it hard to realize that there are several active subprocesses going on (Levelt, 1998). Normal speech involves a sequential process starting with: (1) an intention, followed by (2) determination of a message structure, (3) lexical selection, (4) morphological modulations, (5) a phonetic plan, and (6) a transmission from the phonetic plan into an articulation program.

Some of these subprocesses need to be separately emulated in AAC; the user will need to "find and form" the words (e.g., navigate the device), the graphic symbols, or the manual signs and activate the output (e.g., produce generated speech through the device).

Typical speech is produced at a rate of two to three words a second and up to 200 words a minute. Fast speaking can sometimes reach a speed of 300 words a minute. Levelt (1993) points out that this is possible because formulation and articulation are "underground processes," which are not under conscious control by the speaker. In natural speech, people do not actively think to select the phonemes and the words—it just appears to be a process that runs on its own. It might be counterproductive (i.e., it would slow things down) if speakers would in fact try to control word and phoneme selection.

Levelt's blueprint of the speaker (Figure 2–1) is currently the most prevalent model of the microgenesis of speech, a description of components and processes that are active in running speech. It shows that speakers fluently and speedily perform the following mental operations in a coordinated (partially sequential, partially parallel) way: lexical selection, syntactic planning, and phonological encoding, all while monitoring their own speech.

A Proposed Framework to Understand Access

Note that Levelt's blueprint contains the components of the sender-message-receiver model (see Figure 1–4) that we discussed in Chapter 1. There, we suggested that the sender-message-receiver model could serve as a framework to understand processes (and interventions) in AAC. *Access* can be used as a general term referring to the facilitation of components in the communication process. It both entails factors within the communicator as outside factors that facilitate the exchange of information. When tracing the process from intention to expression and from expression to response by the environment, several key moments can be identified. Most of the typical AAC processes are related to access facilitation (i.e., ways to reinforce, accelerate, circumvent, or provide alternatives for the typical speech processes). Figure 2–2 gives an overview of where in this process some of the AAC techniques and tools can be situated.

Rate of Expressive Communication

The rate of typical speech (200 words a minute) is generally assumed to be commensurate with comfortable information expression and reception. As discussed in the previous chapter, the use of channels other than natural speech, as is often the case in AAC, holds the risk to slow down the speed of conveying strings of words. The slowdown of the utterance speed is a major issue of concern in regards to AAC. The lack of speed can have an impact on:

1. The interaction of cognitive planning and communicative expression.

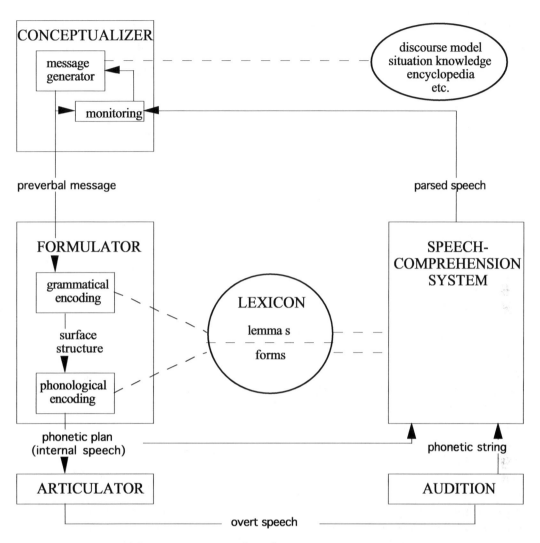

Figure 2–1. Levelt's blueprint of the speaker (1993). Reproduced with permission.

If communication production slows down, the communication partners could start to struggle with short-term memory problems. During speech production of an utterance, speakers know and remember how they start a sentence until the end of the utterance. In typical speech, fragments of the utterance are prepared in the head of the speaker and kept in a "syntactic buffer" waiting to be processed by the phonological encoder (i.e., the part of the message generator that plans the actual speech articulation). In the case of AAC, the waiting time of the planned utterance parts is likely to be increased. The speed of speaking needs to keep pace with the speaker's unfolding of thought. The frustration that this causes may be one of the reasons (not

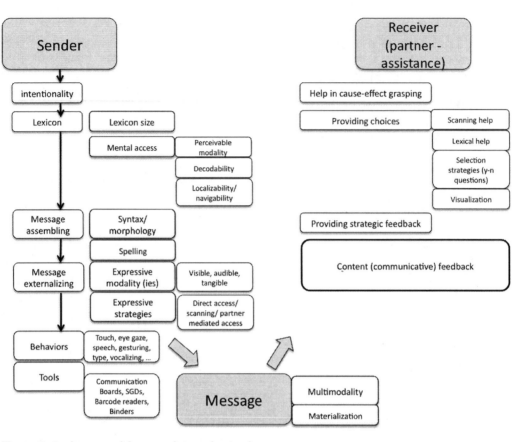

Figure 2–2. A proposed framework to understand access.

the only one) why there is AAC device and AAC system abandonment (i.e., the phenomenon that AAC users and their partners cease to use the system).

2. The trade-off between invested effort (cognitively, linguistically, and physically) and result: because augmented speech requires more effort, speakers may tend to simplify and economize linguistic structure (e.g., dropping morphological endings, limiting the message to key words, and symbols; see also Chapter 7).

3. The willingness and ability of communication partners to participate in the communication exchange: a decreased rate of communication affects all communication partners. Listening to a person who uses AAC may require more attention, patience, and interaction discipline (e.g., waiting your turn) than is needed in communication with typical speakers.

Users of AAC can often not rely on automatically running "underground processes." For example, a person who uses a device needs to locate where in the internal structure of the device the word or message is stored. The efficacy of a device or AAC solution is often measured in the number of keystrokes that are needed to find and activate a word, a symbol, or a prestored message.

ACCESS

The purpose of AAC is to establish or reinforce the connection between the intention to communicate and the actual production of a communicative message through providing alternatives and strategies. These alternatives stem from the two access forms *physical access* and *mental access*.

Physical Access

Physical access is about observable behaviors. Within AAC, we try to find alternatives for the physical production of the message. Instead of natural speech, individuals will point, sign, touch (a screen, a button, a communication board), and use a speech-generating barcode scanner, because these behaviors are more *accessible* to the person. Physical access can imply a sequence of coordinated and planned behaviors: for example, persons might first blink their eyes to indicate the segment of a communication board where the symbol is to be found, after which they use eye blinking to identify one specific symbol on the board. Physical access can also be influenced by seating and positioning (Costigan, 2010) if the person is in a comfortable position and physically able to activate (navigate and operate) a device (or to point, gesture, eye gaze), while maintaining a view of the communication partner and objects of reference in the immediate environment.

Mental Access

Mental access is about internal processes (i.e., about the possibility to mentally conceptualize a message, retrieve a symbol, and plan its utterance). AAC intervention is often geared toward making symbols more mentally accessible. It is about structuring information. For example, many AAC solutions involve some form of *visualization*, a means that sometimes makes it easier for a person to grasp the information (e.g., on a display or board). Another way of improving mental access could be the limitation of available lexical elements. Having fewer words, signs, and/or graphic symbols is often considered to be a disadvantage. However, it may be beneficial in cases where the users are overwhelmed by the sheer number of words (typical language users know tens of thousands of words and usually have little problems in managing them—this may not be the case for some AAC users).

Portability

One of the major ergonomic challenges of aided communication is the *portability*, the possibility to have the solutions available at all times. Can it really be available at all times? Although, miniaturization of devices has increased the portability, sometimes it may not be possible to use a device. Regardless, it is important that AAC users and their communication partners develop a number of *unaided strategies* that will help them establish and maintain communication when the person is in the swimming pool, in a car seat, or simply if the communication device breaks down. One can always fall back to a yes-no question technique. AAC users and their partners should practice this technique. The AAC users answer the question by producing an agreed upon behavior to indicate "yes" or "no" (eye blinking, vocalization, tongue pointing, . . . anything goes as long as it is based on a convention between user and partner). Simple tools can sometimes supplement this, such as a left and right wristband to indicate "yes" or "no" (the user points or stares at the L or R wristband, Figure 2–3).

SENDER ACCESS FACILITATION

Intentionality

Communication is more likely to be effective if the sender has and displays the intention to interact, and acts in order to obtain a response from the communication partner. In typical development, intentionality develops naturally through human interaction during the first months

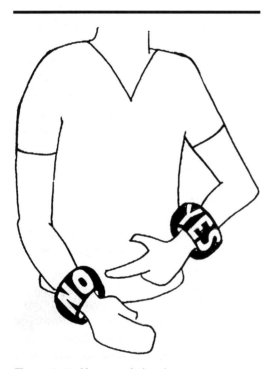

Figure 2–3. Yes-no wristbands.

of life. In individuals with severe developmental limitations, explicit efforts may need to be made to establish a behavioral understanding of a relation between one's own behaviors and responses from others in the environment. The use of AAC tools such as miniatiure objects (tangible symbols) can serve to help evoke this sense of intentionality (see Chapter 6).

Lexicon Accessibility

Within psycholinguistics, the term lexicon is used to refer to the internationalized database of words. Human lexicons contain thousands of entries (called lemmas). The words are internally organized and structured in such a way that easy and quick word retrieval is possible. A typical speaker or listener must be able to "find" (or recognize) the right word within milliseconds. These processes are similar to what AAC users do when they internally select a manual sign, or choose a symbol from a communication board, or find the symbol by navigating through computer pages. As mentioned, the speed of retrieval may be a crucial issue in AAC.

Lexicon Size

Selecting a word in the lexicon implies activation of the lexical item, but at the same time one has to reject competitors. Despite having to deal with an enormous lexicon, most typical language users experience only sporadically problems as a result of one competitor blocking the real word to "come out" (the exception is the "tip of the tongue" phenomenon).

But AAC users may be in a different situation. Could it be that processing will be facilitated if fewer choices are available? Some educators believe that for some (certainly not all) AAC users, "less can be more." In that case, a well-selected small lexicon might be a help (see Chapter 5 for a more extended discussion).

Mental Access to Lexicon

The sender's lexical selection (i.e., the decision which symbols to choose) can be facilitated in a number of ways. Within AAC, this is often done by presenting the person with a preselected and limited number of choices, such as the graphic symbols on communication boards. Symbols also need to be made mentally accessible (i.e., the user needs to be able to retain them and decode them). Often this is done by simply offering them in the visual (rather than auditory) modality. Symbols are easier to access when they can be decoded (e.g., when the user can recognize which parts they are made of). Lexical searches can also be made easier. The better symbols are organized, the easier and faster their retrieval will be. This is obviously the case for any typical lexical access (Levelt, Roelofs, & Meyer, 1999). It is certainly also true for access in AAC. Access can also be facilitated by spatially organizing symbols in a meaningful way on a communication board. For example, nouns and verbs can be assigned specific areas on the display, which would be a linguistic-categorical organization. Often, communication displays are organized in a semantic way (e.g., food items are placed together). If the person is literate, a keyboard (or letter board) is the best possible lay out: as in typing, the person constructs the words with the letters, sometimes aided by word prediction.

Sets and Systems of Symbols: Do They Help in Lexical Access?

Within a natural language, lexicons are systems. The words have a number of organizational principles in common: they are all structured as combinations of a limited number of phonemes (the sounds of the language). Therefore, words can be phonologically decoded. Although the phonemes as such have no meaning, they provide the language user a fast access and a storing system. *Manual signs* are also structured and processed as elements of a system. In fact, linguists talk about the phonology of sign languages, a system of combining a limited number of hand shapes, movements, and body locations. Manual signers benefit from this structural characteristic: they encode, decode, and mentally store signs according to their phonological unique combination (Gutierrez, Williams, Grosvald, & Corina, 2012). However, for graphic symbols, this is not always the case. Many graphic symbols are organized in a *set*, rather than in a *system*. A graphic *symbol set* is a collection of graphic symbols with no clear or well-defined common principle among the symbols (if you make a combination of photographs, pictures copied or cut from magazines, and maybe your own drawings, you have a set—a collection). Graphic *symbol systems* are graphic symbols that are created according to formational and combinatorial rules, in which the same principles are recognizable. Often, combinations of two or more simple symbols represent more complex ideas. Bliss-system (Jennische, 2012; see also Chapter 4) is an example of a well-organized language-like system. The same basic forms are used in different symbols. Symbol systems have something in common with natural languages (i.e., linguistic systems): they share the combinatoriality principle. A limited number of building blocks (a limited number of phonemes) are used to produce an unlimited number of words. For this reason, graphic symbol systems are supposedly appealing to linguistic capacities of the users.

Localizability–Navigability

As mentioned, *portability* is an important consideration. One will need to strike a balance between completeness (having many or all the symbols available) and practicality (weight, time to find the symbols by navigating a device or leafing through the pages of a binder). Therefore, organization of the information in binders and on the communication boards needs to receive careful consideration. *Navigation* though a binder or through a communication device needs to take as little time as possible. One should remember that, in normal communication, a message takes only seconds to produce. The challenge of AAC is to keep the communication as natural (in speed) as possible, in order to achieve effectiveness and minimize frustration (both in the communicator and in the partner) as well as avoid AAC abandonment.

Navigation with MinSpeak

Most of the devices allow you to organize messages on screens in a size and format that can be modified by the users or their assistants. In most cases, users will have to navigate through the pages (called the dynamic displays—as one button often opens a new screen) to identify the symbol or the message that they need. The storage capacity of these devices is virtually unlimited—the problem is the

navigation and the speed of access. One solution for the navigation problem is the use of the Minspeak code, developed by Bruce Baker (2012). Minspeak is a combination of symbols (called icons) that, for the most part, do not represent direct meanings. A combination code generates meanings. For example, for "I love coffee" you will need to hit the "I" icon twice, then the LOVE icon (illustrating a mother holding a baby), followed by the MR. ACTION MAN, verb icon (illustrating worker with bucket and hammer), and finally the DRINK button, followed by the COFFEE button in the activity row. This system may be less intuitive at first sight, but it allows the user to stay away from navigation and proceed faster (Figure 2–4).

From a cognitive processing point of view, navigation requires time and memory (knowing where the message is stored). Icon sequencing (such as Minspeak) requires the person initially to remember the "code." Proponents of the Minspeak system believe that this is mainly a process of motor learning and motor memory—comparable with what individuals "know" about a computer keyboard. Many keyboard users may not be able to answer if you ask them "where is the 'g' on the keyboard," but they may be fast and flawless when they have to type a word that contains a "g."

In recent years, a number of authors (Center for AAC and Autism, 2009) have suggested that "language acquisition through motor planning" (or LAMP) is what is needed. Producing symbol sequences could be compared with the complex motor patterns of natural speech (Browman & Goldstein, 1990), except that augmented communicators are using symbols to construct messages. Fluent communication on an AAC device is

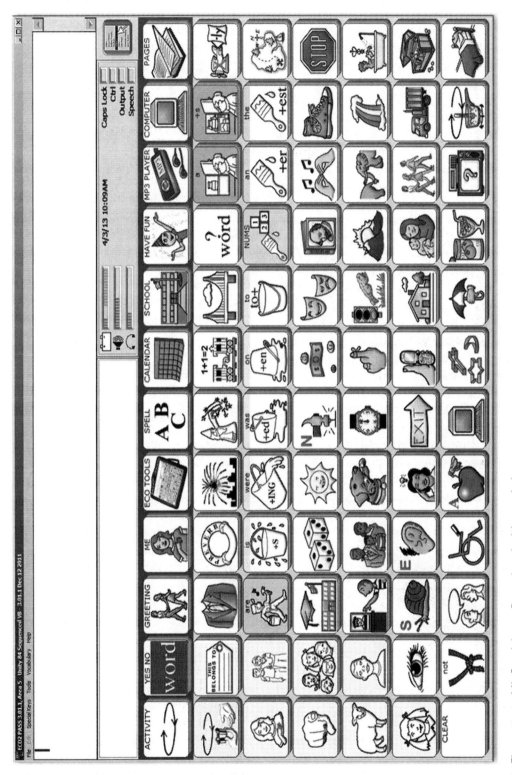

Figure 2–4. MinSpeak icons. Reproduced with permission.

facilitated by learned and repetitive patterns that have become automatized. Constructing messages using the LAMP approach is also an assembly process that requires the communicator to sequence a series of choices and actions. In many ways, this is similar to the morphological and syntactical planning and execution in typical speech, although it can have its specific characteristics in AAC. For example, the use of Minspeak requires a unique serial combination of icons (icon sequencing), an operation that does not have a direct equivalent in typical speech production. The production of syntactic sequences is a different process in AAC because the assembly and production process typically takes more time, which can lead to a discrepancy between planning time (thinking of the utterance to express) and execution time. One challenge and a matter of debate of the system is its learnability by young children (Drager & Light, 2010). In order to study how the system is best acquired by young children, a methodology will be needed that focuses on the acquisition of coding rules, not single words and meanings.

Access to Message Assembly Techniques

Syntax and Morphology Techniques (Prestored Phrases)

Syntax and morphology of a message often may have to be sacrificed to meet requirements of speed in the conversation. It can also be a result of syntactic memory limitations. One solution that is used in AAC software is prestored phrases and messages.

Spelling (Word Prediction) and Keystroke Economy

Navigation and search for a prestored message within a device can be facilitated by minimizing the number of keystrokes, and by making the search pattern analogous (Higginbotham, 1992). Keystroke saving becomes possible through the use of word prediction *software*, a feature that is now commonly available and daily used in mobile computing and other mainstream applications (Trnka, McCraw, Yarrington, McCoy, & Pennington, 2008). Word prediction systems make it possible to accelerate the speed of AAC expression, as long as the method is using word typing (and as long as the user is literate).

Message Externalizing

Selection of Accessible Modality

Visual Modality. Graphic symbols—including object symbols—can and should be used to visualize information in schedules, calendars, almanacs, activity sheets, and so on. This reminds us of two things: (1) we use language and symbols not only for communication—but also to guide and structure our thinking. When AAC is provided, a person's communication is not only supported, but also their life's functionality; (2) for many people, visualization is an important channel to process information. A majority of AAC tools contain a visual aspect. Although the product of natural speech is hard to grasp, the acoustic flow is dynamic and changes as a function of time—visual information is often more static and allows for longer processing time. We use graphic symbols on paper, on flash cards, on communication boards, and on the screen displays of communication devices. Manual signs, frequently used by nonspeaking individuals with intellectual disabilities, are also visually represented. While they are not static, the visual impression lasts longer than the acoustic signal of the spoken word. Visually processing a manual sign may be easier than processing a spoken word. This is one of the explanations why manual signing sometimes works for people with developmental challenges.

Audible Modality. Speech is the most prevalent communication system that uses the audible modality. Most AAC practices include the parallel (simultaneous) use of speech with other modalities. Communication partners are generally encouraged to produce speech together with the alternative forms, and many of the communication systems do have (often synthetic) speech output.

Tangible Modality. Individuals functioning at the sensori-motor interaction level as well as persons with visual impairment can benefit from the presence of tactile information, usually in the form of tangible symbols (including small objects that are passed between sender and receiver).

Expressive Strategies

Direct Access. We talk about *direct activation* when a user has direct control over and access to the communication tool that is used, and when the operation is primarily guided by the communicator. For example, the user touches a field on a screen, which generates the speech by the device. Note that unaided communication always implies the use of direct activation (in the case of natural speech or manual

signing, activation can be considered to be an internal process.)

In most cases, a selection process precedes activation.

Scanning. The environment can provide other ways of facilitating selection. This is often done through *scanning*. Scanning is sequentially presenting stimuli (or categories of stimuli) to which the person can respond. Responding entails activation. For example, several choices of graphic symbols may sequentially light up on a communication screen, allowing the user to physically respond (e.g., by activating a switch) to the desired stimulus.

Behavior

Which behavior do AAC users observably produce? This includes the "alternative" forms that give AAC its most visible characteristics: eye gazing, pointing, gesturing, touching a communication screen, and so on. In a way, this is not different from typical communication, although one single form of communication may carry most of the information (speech is the main information carrier in typical communication), in reality several forms are often used together (gestures, pointing, eye gaze, vocal interjections).

Vocalizing/Speech

By definition, most AAC users have limited use of functional speech, but that doesn't mean that no speech is used. The use of alternative forms often simultaneously triggers some speech (see Chapter 10). Vocalizations (the production of vocal sound) do not need to be speech (i.e., spoken word production) but they can indicate specific meanings (often only understood by familiar partners).

Eye Gaze

The person builds a message by sequentially looking at and fixating at an element on a communication device (nontech or tech) or directly at an object. Eye-gaze technology is software connected with a camera and a computer. It converts eye gaze steering into computer actions. Such a set up enables voice output and steering a computer (Chapter 3).

Gesturing

Gestures are movements of the arms and body that can be used as communicative expressive behaviors. They can also be idiosyncratic behaviors that are only recognized by familiar communication partners for their communicative value. They can also be more conventionalized forms of gesturing (see Chapter 4), as is the case for manual signs that have a linguistic nature (e.g., signs borrowed from an existing sign language, or signs "designed" for AAC purposes). A special form of gesturing is pointing, which developmentally emerges from grasping and reaching (Delgado, Gómez, & Sarriá, 2011), and which serves important prelinguistic functions such as labeling. *Manual signs* are gestures that have become conventionalized within a linguistic system (e.g., in a sign language).

Touching

Touching is used in many AAC applications to indicate or activate (e.g., in the case of a switch or a speech generating device) a chosen message or symbol. It is often related to pointing. Touching is one of the most used direct access methods.

Typing

Typing is composing words and messages by using a real or virtual (on-screen) keyboard. Typing employs an orthographic spelling system (e.g., the English alphabet) to produce a written message on a screen or paper.

Brain Activity

The possibilities of access are dramatically increasing as new and more advanced technologies are developed. According to some, the ongoing research into Brain-Computer Interaction (BCI) will, probably within the next few years, become more mainstream and available for persons with severe paralysis. Through BCI, a person learns to send signals through brainwave sensors to a computer screen. By doing this, the person controls the computer and can send messages or do other operations. Much research still needs to be done, but the groundwork for these innovations are laid (Thompson, Blain-Moraes, & Huggins, 2013). This is a major step forward toward liberating people with the so-called Locked-in syndrome, a condition in which a person is left with almost no voluntary body movements, while retaining normal cognitive functions.

Tools

Speech Generating Devices

Speech generating devices (SGD) is the name currently used for devices that have synthetic or digitized speech output. SGDs can be simple (containing a limited number of prestored messages) or advanced (allowing generation of an infinite number of novel speech utterances/ allowing organizing the messages in electronic pages and grids). SGDs can allow the generated speech to be connected with other electronic applications (including internet access and general use software packages). SGDs can function as dedicated devices (solely serving communication) or integrated into computers, tablets, or cell phones (mobile computing; see Chapter 3).

Barcode Reader

Barcode reading technology combined with digitized or synthetic speech can be used in devices that recognize barcodes. Barcodes can be attached to objects, pictures, clothes, schedules, and more (Loncke, Alves, & Meyer, 2006) (see also Figure 8–2).

Communication Boards (and Symbol Displays)

Communication boards and symbol displays are among the oldest and most used AAC tools. They come in nontech, low-tech, and high-tech forms. The essential characteristic is that users have a visual display from which they select symbols. The symbols can be organized in grids (different sizes, hence different number of symbols to choose from) or arranged in other ways (e.g., in a thematic visual scene). The most effective organization is dependent on processing abilities and strengths of the users (Wilkinson & Light, 2011).

One can also use a simple letter board. The letters on the board can be organized in any configuration, depending on the skills and preferences of the user and the partners (abc—order, keyboard configuration, in combination with short phrases, and so on).

Tactile Symbols

Tangible or tactile symbols are (usually small) objects that can be held in the hands, shown to a communication partner, and handed over as a communicative act. These symbols can serve two functions. First, they can be used as a form of object communication (making the communication act a "materialized" and concrete event). This is especially helpful for individuals who function at a basic communicative level (Rowland, Schweigert, & Educational Resources Information Center, 1991). Second, deaf-blind individuals can use the symbols. People with dual sensory impairment can indeed benefit from the tangibly recognizable features (Lund & Troha, 2008).

Switches

Switches (see Figure 3–2) are powerful tools within assistive technology. Through switches, a complex activity is reduced to a single-movement response that may be repeated several times according to the schema of action. For example, a device that has a grid display (columns and rows) can first light up row-by-row, which allows the switch user to click when the desired row is highlighted (see scanning). Subsequently the device will light up the columns (from left to right), and the user clicks when the targeted symbol is reached (see Chapter 3).

Other Tools and Devices

Increasingly, communication symbols and external aids to communication are stored and accessed in nondedicated formats (i.e., tools that were initially not designed to be used for augmentative communication). These can be nontech materials such as binders, small etch-and-sketch boards, besides desktop, laptop computers, or mobile computing platforms (such as iPhones and tablets) containing symbol software besides other applications (Bradshaw & Bradshaw, 2013; also see Chapter 3). Newer developments go in the direction of making tools (or some components of them) virtual by storing information (e.g., symbol representations) as part of Cloud computing.

MESSAGE TRANSMISSION

In typical communication, the transmission of the message is fast and essentially invisible. Nobody can see the words flow from the sender to the receiver. AAC includes techniques to make this transmission more explicit, more concrete, and enhanced.

Multimodality Principle

One of the most salient characteristics of AAC is that expressive modalities are chosen that are different from predominantly speech-only. The behaviors that form the communicative act can include gestures, pointing, eye gazing, vocalizing, and any behavior that can serve as a device activator (e.g., tongue movements, head movements, elbow movements, eye movements). AAC may require transitive movements (i.e., movements that are executed on external objects such as a communication board or a communica-

tion device). This requires special coordination skills.

An example of AAC use at the level of message transition is the practice of simultaneous communication (e.g., the use of speech and manual signing in a synchronized way; Whitehead, Schiavetti, Whitehead, & Metz, 1997). The purpose of this practice is to establish a mutual reinforcement of signal in different modes (e.g., one says "let's go to the house" and signs GO— HOUSE parallel to the spoken message).

Materialization Principle

Transmission of the message can be facilitated in a number of ways. One obvious way is through materialization of the symbols, using them as objects that can be manipulated and physically exchanged between communication partners (Figure 2–5). The PECS system is an excellent example of this principle (Bondy & Frost, 1994). *Object communication* is an attempt to help individuals to understand that symbols are referents—they refer to things (or to actions, or concepts). In object communication, you intensify the relation between the symbol and the referent. In fact, the symbol looks a lot like the referent as it is an object.

Note that Figure 2–5, besides being an example of object communication, is also an example of multimodality. Several representations of the same referent are united—the miniature object, the picture (the graphic symbol), and the printed word (Traditional Orthography, or TO). In its daily use, you will probably speak while you are handling these object symbols, adding the *spoken modality* to the whole configuration of modalities.

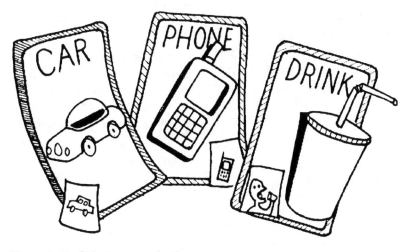

Figure 2–5. Object communication.

THE RECEIVER'S ROLE AND ASSISTANCE FROM COMMUNICATION PARTNER

The communication partner can do several things to facilitate the process. By providing strategic feedback, the partner helps the communicator to make lexical choices and progress through an utterance and/or a conversation. Many of the strategies in AAC are not directly activated, but are the result of *co-construction*, also known as *partner-assisted communication*. This blurs the clear distinction between sender and receiver—as the receiver takes over some of the tasks of the sender. Sender and receiver work together on the construction of the message. For example, if the receiver asks yes-no questions, it will reduce the sender's efforts (to a simple movement) and will speed up the conversation. Partner-assisted communication is an attempt to reduce the "costs" of communication (the physical effort, the time investment, the risks of misunderstanding).

Help in the Physical Execution of the Message

Partners can help the person in the physical execution of the message (e.g., by molding the manual signs that is appropriate, or by holding the hand toward a letter board, or a keyboard). The latter is a technique that has been proposed by proponents of *facilitated communication* (FC), who suggest that some individuals will be able to express their thoughts if they get some minimal physical support by a (physical) facilitator. Since the mid 1990s when the technique was first introduced, discussion and controversy about this method has been going on. The debate centered on the question whether the outcomes of FC interactions were more the result of overinterpretation by the facilitator (the communication partner) and not a genuine reflection of the authorship by the person. The discussion between strong defenders and proponents (Biklen & Schneiderman, 1997; Crossley, 1997) and more skeptical researchers (Regal & Rooney, 1994) continues to this day.

Help in Cause–Effect Grasping

Individuals with severe intellectual disabilities may need help in distinguishing cause and effect, and grasping their relation. This can be part of an individual educational program (IEP). Typically, this is done by systematically exposing the person to the same or similar sequences of events that will help the person to recognize a temporal (predictive) relation. In particular, it is most effective in shaping behaviors toward requesting or rejecting items (Choi, O'Reilly, Sigafoos, & Lancioni, 2010). Cause-effect grasping facilitates the development of intentionality.

Providing Choices

An obvious example of partner help is the communication partner *offering choices*. The communication partner may verbally ask "coffee" or "tea," narrowing down the possibilities, while at the same time allowing the person to indicate the preferred stimulus by an easily interpreted response (e.g., head nodding, blinking, smiling). Visual aids (e.g., in the form of a simple communication board) can help individuals to make decisions (Bailey, Willner, & Dymond, 2011).

Help with Scanning

The user will then point or gaze in a direction—or, in partner-assisted communication, the partner points at blocks and letters on the board. Figure 2–6 shows an Etran (from Eye-Transfer) eye-gaze board with graphic symbols where the two communication partners are facing each other. The transparent board is an open frame

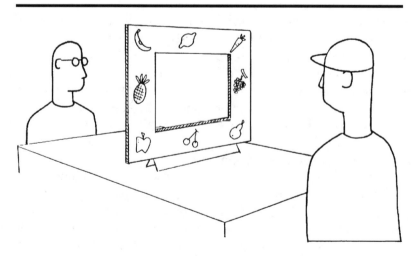

Figure 2–6. Eye-gaze graphic symbol board.

through which the communication partner can see the direction in which the person is gazing (to indicate the symbol of choice). Figure 2–7 shows the same screen with letter blocks.

One can also work with an "imaginary letter board." In this case, the user and partner are an experienced team who understand each other enough that the AAC user knows to indicate yes or no if the partner says A-block, or G-block, and so on. Eye-gaze based letter boards are sometimes used in communication with a nonspeaking person in a hospital bed.

The board is held between patient (AAC user) and caregiver. The caregiver looks through the hole in the middle and determines which block the person is looking at. The caregiver may think the person is looking at the RSTUV block. (Note that the two sides have a mirror-image configuration.) If the patient looks at the block left under, it will be the block right under for the partner. The partner asks, "Do you want the R-block?"—the patient blinks once (yes) or twice (no). If yes, the partner

will say R-S-T-U-V. The patient blinks at the moment that the desired letter is said. Then, the partner continues to find the second letter, and so on.

Lexical Help

Each time an AAC user is provided with a display with graphic symbols that are considered to be helpful in a specific situation (e.g., the store, breakfast, a medical exam), lexical help is provided. The board facilitates quick selection without much navigation. However, preselected symbols (or phrases) can at the same time be a limitation for the user as they restrict the scope of topics, questions, responses, and comments that can be made.

Selection Strategies (Y–N Questions)

In the popular game "21 Questions," one participant tries to find a word by solely asking yes-no questions. Clever players

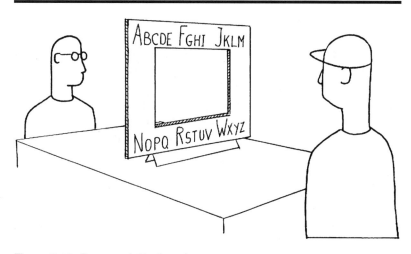

Figure 2–7. Eye-gaze letter board.

know how to ask questions in an economic way (i.e., by limiting the number of questions before the answer if found). Exactly the same simple but powerful principle can be used in AAC, where the AAC users can indicate "yes" or "no" with an agreed upon behavior.

Visualization

Many AAC applications not only provide visually accessible symbols (graphic symbols, manual signs) but also include ways in which these symbols are organized. Symbols can be organized in calendars, task schedules, thematic pages, or thematic visual scenes. The lay out of graphic symbols on a board or a display can help the person to accelerate choice making, to better see the relation between elements, or to get a perspective on a hierarchical relation between concepts and ideas.

Joan Murphy, a Scottish speech-language pathologist, conceived and developed "Talking Mats," a communication tool that consists of a mat that can be spread between the person with communication limitations and a communication partner. The mat is used to display graphic symbols (or objects) in a spatial arrangement that helps the communicators to view the relation between objects, persons, events, and ideas (Figure 2–8). A conversation can be accompanied by: grouping the symbols together, placing them in opposite locations, removing them, adding them, or otherwise changing the spatial relationship. This low-tech tool allows a dynamic ongoing visualization of the evolving ideas. This approach has shown to be helpful for people with intellectual and cognitive limitations (Murphy & Boa, 2012).

Strategic Feedback

Strategic feedback refers to what the communication partner does to facilitate how the AAC user organizes the execution of the message. For example, the communication partner can ask, "Do you find what you have to say on the page?," "Can you reach to the board?," and "Would you like me to read the list?"

Content Feedback

Content feedback occurs when the communication partner checks if the message is well-interpreted and understood. The communication partner can say something like, "I think you just said you don't want to stay here any longer," or "am I correct, did you just say that . . . ?" Communication partners need to develop the skill to interpret and provide feedback, without overinterpreting what the AAC users just said. The appropriateness of both strategic and content feedback is highly dependent on the level of trust and comfort between AAC user and communication partner.

POINTS TO REMEMBER

■ Success of AAC is dependent not only on the user but also on the communication partner (e.g., there must be strategic feedback and content feedback).

■ Most of the typical AAC processes are related to facilitation of access (i.e., ways to reinforce, accelerate, circumvent, or provide alternatives for typical speech processes).

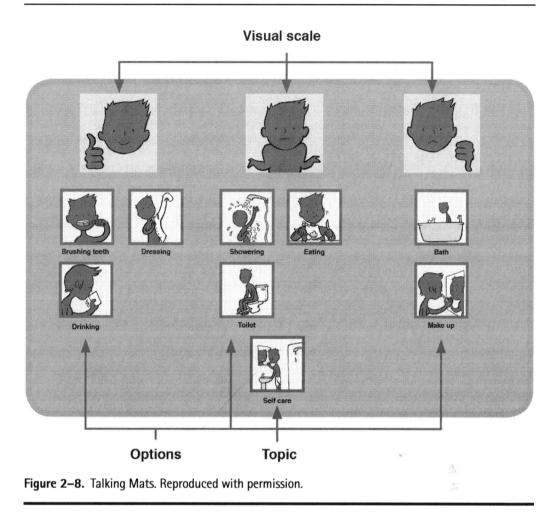

Figure 2–8. Talking Mats. Reproduced with permission.

- To understand AAC, it is necessary to pay attention to mental processes like word/symbol retrieval, combination of symbols, and short-term memory management.
- The AAC user uses intentionality, lexicon, message assembling, message externalizing, behaviors, and tools to communicate the message to the receiver, who helps with cause-effect grasping, providing choices, and providing strategic feedback.
- Mental access involves the conceptualization of the message, retrieval of the symbol, and planning of the utterance. It is the internal act of planning the message or the intention. Physical access is the actual behavior required to convey the planned message. It is a sequence of coordinated and planned behaviors.
- Access facilitation includes ways to reinforce, accelerate, circumvent, and/or provide alternatives for the typical speech process. AAC combines both physical access (behaviors) and mental access (internal processes) as alternative strategies to communicate.

■ Symbols and messages can be found through different strategies (e.g., through screen navigation or through icon sequencing). Both strategies rely on different processes.

REFERENCES

Bailey, R., Willner, P., & Dymond, S. (2011). A visual aid to decision-making for people with intellectual disabilities. *Research in Developmental Disabilities, 32*(1), 37–46.

Baker, B. (2012). *How Minspeak allows for independent communication by giving anyone access to core vocabulary.* Message posted to http://www.minspeak.com/CoreVocabulary.php

Biklen, D., & Schneiderman, H. (1997). Facilitated communication. *Pediatrics, 99*(2), 308–309.

Bondy, A. S., & Frost, L. A. (1994). The picture exchange communication system. *Focus on Autistic Behavior, 9*(3), 1–19.

Bradshaw, J., & Bradshaw, J. (2013). The use of augmentative and alternative communication apps for the iPad, iPod and iPhone: An overview of recent developments. *Tizard Learning Disability Review, 18*(1), 31–37.

Browman, C. P., & Goldstein, L. (1990). Gestural specification using dynamically-defined articulatory structures. *Journal of Phonetics, 18*(3), 299–320.

Center for AAC and Autism. (2009). *What is LAMP? (language acquisition through motor planning).* Retrieved from http://www.aacandautism.com/lamp

Choi, H., O'Reilly, M., Sigafoos, J., & Lancioni, G. (2010). Teaching requesting and rejecting sequences to four children with developmental disabilities using augmentative and alternative communication. *Research in Developmental Disabilities, 31*(2), 560–567.

Costigan, F. A. (2010). Effect of seated position on upper-extremity access to augmentative communication for children with cerebral palsy: Preliminary investigation. *The American Journal of Occupational Therapy, 64*(4), 596.

Crossley, R. (1997). *Speechless. Facilitating communication for people without voices.* New York, NY: Dutton/ Penguin Group.

Delgado, B., Gómez, J. C., & Sarriá, E. (2011). Pointing gestures as a cognitive tool in young children: Experimental evidence. *Journal of Experimental Child Psychology, 110*(3), 299–312.

Drager, K. D. R., & Light, J. C. (2010). A comparison of the performance of 5-year-old children with typical development using iconic encoding in AAC systems with and without icon prediction on a fixed display. *Augmentative and Alternative Communication, 26*(1), 12–20.

Gutierrez, E., Williams, D., Grosvald, M., & Corina, D. (2012). Lexical access in American Sign Language: An ERP investigation of effects of semantics and phonology. *Brain Research, 1468*(0), 63–83.

Higginbotham, D. J. (1992). Evaluation of keystroke savings across five assistive communication technologies. *Augmentative and Alternative Communication, 8*(4), 258–272.

Jennische, M. (2012). *Characteristics of Blissymbolics.* Presentation at the International Society for augmentative and alternative communi-cation research seminar. Pittsburgh, Pennsylvania.

Levelt, W. J. M. (1993). *Speaking: From intention to articulation* (1st MIT Pbk. ed.). Cambridge, MA: MIT Press.

Levelt, W. J. M. (1998). The genetic perspective in psycholinguistics or where do spoken words come from? *Journal of Psycholinguistic Research, 27*(2), 167–180.

Levelt, W. J. M., Roelofs, A., & Meyer, A. S. (1999). A theory of lexical access in speech production. *Behavioral and Brain Sciences, 22*(1), 1–38.

Loncke, F., Alves, M., & Meyer, L. (2006). B.A.bar: The speaking barcode reader. *Closing the Gap,* 21–22.

Lund, S. K., & Troha, J. M. (2008). Teaching young people who are blind and have autism to make requests using a variation on the picture exchange communication system with tactile symbols: A preliminary investigation. *Journal of Autism and Developmental Disorders, 38*(4), 719–730.

Murphy, J., & Boa, S. (2012). Using the WHO-ICF with talking mats to enable adults with long-term communication difficulties to participate in goal setting. *AAC: Augmentative and Alternative Communication, 28*(1), 52–60 (60 ref).

Regal, R. A., & Rooney, J. R. (1994). Facilitated communication: An experimental evaluation.

Journal of Autism and Developmental Disorders, 24(3), 345–355.

Rowland, C., Schweigert, P., & Educational Resources Information Center. (1991, 1990). *Tangible symbol systems.* Tucson, AZ: Communication Skill Builders.

Thompson, D., Blain-Moraes, S., & Huggins, J. (2013). Performance assessment in brain-computer interface-based augmentative and alternative communication. *BioMedical Engineering OnLine, 12*(1), 43.

Trnka, K., McCraw, J., Yarrington, D., McCoy, K., & Pennington, C. (2008). Word prediction and communication rate in AAC. *Proceedings of the IASTED International Conference on Assistive Technologies—AT2008* (pp. 19–24). Baltimore, MD.

Whitehead, R. L., Schiavetti, N., Whitehead, B. H., & Metz, D. E. (1997). Effect of sign task on speech timing in simultaneous communication. *Journal of Communication Disorders, 30*(6), 439–455.

Wilkinson, K. M., & Light, J. (2011). Preliminary investigation of visual attention to human figures in photographs: Potential considerations for the design of aided AAC visual scene displays. *Journal of Speech, Language, and Hearing Research, 54*(6), 1644–1657.

CHAPTER 3

Nontech, Low-Tech, High-Tech, and Mobile Computing

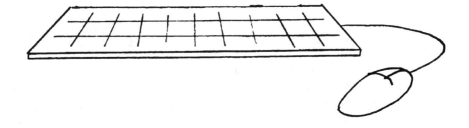

The two words of "assistive technology" are equally important. It is "technology"—the use of techniques, materials, and tools to improve an individual's functioning in the world. However, it is also "assistive," its use—or at least its introduction—needs to have a component of helping, teaching (training if you will) in order to make sure that the clients are integrating its use in their daily functioning. This requires information, training, modeling, counseling, and feedback. In other words, one doesn't just hand over the device (or tell them what the technique consists of) and expect that the clients (and their communication and life partners) will adopt it without any problem.

Within the field of AAC, the scope of choices has grown intensively. When should we use nontech approaches and when is high-tech (and everything in the middle) more appropriate? Very often, the range of devices and methods that exist within AAC overwhelms the practitioner. Clinicians frequently express uncertainty about their own knowledge of the field and the choices, and fear that they might not make the best decisions and recommendations. It is true that, with the general rapid development of information and communication technology (computers, miniaturization, and mobile computing), newer AAC devices become available every year, if not every month. Not only are there new devices, but applications (within the device) expand. From 2005 on, more models and types of AAC devices have been integrated within a computer platform—which enables the user in principle to integrate communication in other applications such as word processing and internet surfing. There are many applications possible and imaginable that imply a combination of direct message production (e.g., access symbols on a screen) with calling up pictures of photographs, films, websites, prestored texts, and more. The more a person can integrate multiple functions, the more likely it is that communication will be effective and really interactive.

ASSISTIVE TECHNOLOGY

Assistive technology (AT) is the term used to indicate technological measures taken to facilitate a person's functioning. It is clear that AT plays an important role within AAC. The augmentation and the alternatives for the typical forms of communication often come from technology. AT can fulfill major contributions to AAC. In order to appreciate the contribution of AT, it is again helpful to take a look at the communication process and identify which components in the process can potentially benefit from AT. Figure 3–1 is an elaboration of Levelt's blueprint of the speaker (see Figure 2–1, Chapter 2) with indications where technology can play a role.

NONTECH, LOW–TECH, AND HIGH–TECH

The term "high-tech" is sometimes used to refer to the "higher end" AAC communication solutions, while "low-tech" is reserved to materials or systems that are "inexpensive, simple and easy to obtain" (Cook & Hussey, 1995, mentioned in Quist & Lloyd, 1997, p. 107). One of the fascinating phenomena of our times has been the increasing possibilities and presence in daily lives of electronic communication, in an ever faster, more flexible, more miniaturized, and accessible way.

Given the rate at which new technologies continue to become available, at reduced costs, often more miniaturized than in previous versions (allowing them to be used as handheld devices), terms like "high" and "low" technology are increasingly relative and should be considered on a dynamic continuum. We do not use this dichotomy, but rather focus on which functions, components, and processes within communication can be technologically supported.

STEERING TECHNOLOGY

For assistive technology, it is important to identify an interface that allows the user to direct a device. Devices are steered by (often a combination of) vision, audition, or touch (Karray, Alemzadeh, Abou Saleh, & Nours Arab, 2008). Vision-based (think of computer or device screens) devices are most often steered by a *switch-based input system*. Traditional keyboards are in fact structures that contain a set of switches. Within AAC and assistive technology, the steering can be reduced to the use of a single switch (or a combined use of a two or a few switches) that is connected with a computer (Figure 3–2).

Pointing-based input systems include the use of a mouse, a joystick, touchscreens, graphic tablets, and pen-based input forms. *Audition-based input systems* have become more prevalent as speech recognition technology has improved. Finally, *haptic input systems* respond to skin and muscle pressure (Ricciardi et al., 2010). Today's steering technology also includes *gestural steering* (Walkowski, Dörner, Lievonen, & Rosenberg, 2011) including the possibility to use manual signs to direct a computer (Jalab, 2012).

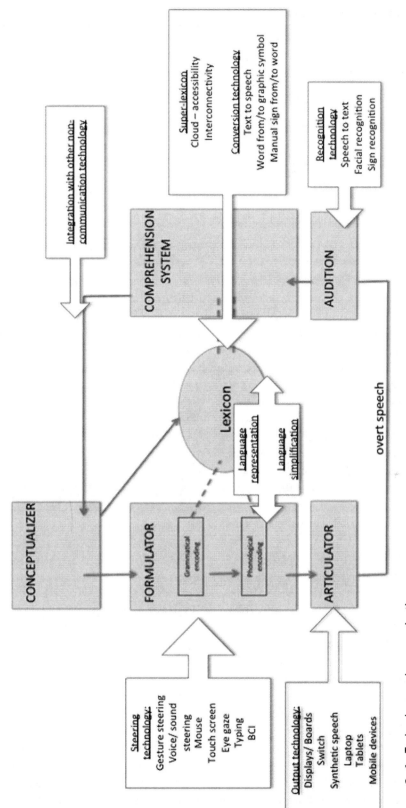

Figure 3–1. Technology and communication.

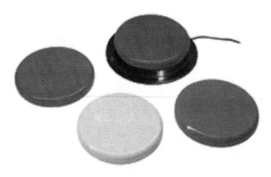

Figure 3–2. Big Red Twist—used with permission from Ablenet.

In the past 15 years, *eye-gaze steering* has developed from cutting edge applications to more affordable and relatively reliable systems used by a growing number of persons with limited mobility. Eye-track devices have been developed for a wide range of purposes, and AAC is just one of the applications. There is a strong interest from psychologists, especially as it provides a way to test the hypothesis that there is a strong connection between what a person focuses on and internal mental processes. This is sometimes called the "strong eye-mind hypothesis" (Just & Just, 1980). Eye tracking research has found applications in automobile driver security research (what are drivers looking at?), machine operation security (do people see what they should see when they are operating a machine?) and locomotion (walking—do older and younger walkers see where they put their feet? Do they notice and pay attention to barriers?), and—of course—the use of your eyes to direct a computer. Today, the systems are readily employed by a growing number of individuals with AAC needs and extremely limited mobility. The costs for the devices have come down, the technology has improved, the learnability has become less demanding, and the weight and size of the devices have been reduced.

Brain-computer interaction, also called direct neural interface or brain-machine interface, is now rapidly developing into a major group of applications within the field of "neuroprosthetics" (2013). Neuroprosthetics is the discipline that searches for substitutions for impaired motor, sensory, and cognitive functions through the use of a device that is controlled and directed by internal body operations. Possibly the best known neuroprosthetic device is a cochlear implant. The newer additions to neuroprosthetics are devices that are controlled by vision and brain activity. We already have studies that show that it is possible to command a computer by BCI and execute computer-generated speech. The applications for AAC continue to be very promising (Thompson, Blain-Moraes, & Huggins, 2013).

LANGUAGE REPRESENTATION TECHNOLOGY

Devices and tools can be used to help a user gain insight in language structure, or access words, letters, phrases, or semantic concepts. However, this implies that devices represent language at some level(s). A traditional typewriter or computer keyboard represents language at the phonological-orthographic level (i.e., by displaying the letters of the alphabet together with punctuation). It requires the users to go from there and put words, phrases, and sentences together, based on their spelling skills. The traditional keyboard is certainly highly generative: It allows the user to produce all possible linguistic combinations. Many AAC devices come with the traditional keyboard, which is indeed often the preferred choice for all who possess spelling and composition skills (see Figure 5–1). However, most AAC displays typically show graphic symbols in some organization. In many applications, the graphic symbols are used as lexical units having single or multiple meanings. Developers of AAC software and their applications suggest generative uses of these lexical graphic items in such a way that they emulate typical generative linguistic use. For example, Van Tatenhoven (2005) proposes strategies for clinicians to enhance and stimulate a child's use and gradual expansion of linguistic functions in increasingly complex syntactic forms.

The way devices present and organize linguistic elements can facilitate specific uses: how fast and easy it is to "find" a symbol, combine it with other symbols, and express simple and complex combinations. MinSpeak is constructed to reinforce the development of a psychomotor-based (motor planning, see: Center for AAC and Autism, 2009) learning of linguistic units (words) by acquiring a code, partially based on an understanding of semantic networks (see also Chapter 2, including Figure 2–4). There are a number of derived applied programs that are focused on facilitating linguistic aspects of language (e.g., Unity, a set of MAPs, or Minspeak Application Programs; Semantic Compaction Systems). Implicitly, most of language representation software are applications of *computational linguistics*, the (mainly applied) discipline that explores how linguistic structures and linguistic behavior (especially word finding and sentence planning) can be emulated by computer software (Vetulani, 2011). In many applications, an algorithm accumulates preferred words, phrases, and structures by a person, accelerating the rate at which probable choices are proposed and can be activated.

WordPower is primarily a word-based system, developed by Nancy Inman. Users work from a limited lexicon of 100 core words that can be accessed and combined fast and easily in order to generate unique messages. Word access is facilitated through semantic organization and clustering that is based on the Fitzgerald Key. The FK is a visualization of syntactic patterns originally proposed by Edith Fitzgerald in 1929 to help deaf children recognize and structure syntactic patterns (Fitzgerald, 1969, 1949). WordPower uses this pattern-principle, together with word prediction and spelling software (Inman, 2013).

Gateway is a system developed by Joan Bruno to be used on dynamic display devices (i.e., devices that allow a user to navigate from screen to screen; from page to page). The system is also word-based. Core words can be accessed with a minimal number of keystrokes. The pages are targeted for different cognitive-linguistic developmental levels, in order to foster communicative-linguistic development (Bruno, 2013).

Proloquo2Go is a graphic symbols word program developed for use on tablets and mobile computing platforms. It combines graphic symbols with printed and device-generated speech output. It allows quick access to core words (Assistiveware, 2013; Hager, 2012).

Boardmaker is software that allows the construction of learning materials, communication boards, behavior supports, and other visualizations of Picture Communication Symbols (PCS; Mayer-Johnson, 2013).

The *Lingraphica* program was developed to be a therapy and communication tool for individuals with acquired language impairments such as aphasia (Steele, Aftonomos, & Koul, 2010). Lingraphica uses graphic symbols that help to identify vocabulary. It also contains syntax patterns that help the user to build sentences.

It is clear that most of the programs are primarily lexicon-based: users identify words, which are associated in networks with other words. Most of the programs associate words in semantic networks, and several provide syntactic cues (such as grouping verbs and nouns together).

OUTPUT TECHNOLOGY

Which material tools do users have to express their message? Obviously, we are talking about *aided communication* (see Chapter 1), because output technology implies the use of tools external to the communicator's body. Some authors have suggested that aided communication can sometimes distract from interpersonal contact. For example, the communication partner might neglect to seek face-to-face contact (hence missing the facial expression cues of the AAC user) and focus on the aid display to which the user is pointing. However, in the past few years, mobile computing has made the use of (electronic) aids so prevalent in the community (not just by and for AAC users) that combined face-to-face and display-focused strategies are now more becoming the rule as they are employed by the general population. Moreover, the miniaturization of cell phones and devices has had for effect that they almost function as an extension to some people's body.

Nontech Output

Sometimes the simplest adaptations provide excellent output forms. In fact, a majority of users of advanced technology solutions also use simple nontech tools, such as letter boards, picture boards or binders, or cards with printed symbols or messages (as in Picture Exchange Communication System).

Furthermore, there are, for example, great possibilities of partner-assisted communication. The AAC user can point to a symbol or message with the finger, with a laser pointer, or with eye gaze, and the partner will facilitate the scanning and selection process by asking questions. The transmission between communicator and partner can benefit from strategic positioning and setup of the communication aids. For early communicators, you could simply put concrete symbols in the visual field between the sender and the receiver by using a communication vest (Figure 3–3).

Device–Generated Speech

There is a wide range of speech generating *electronic communication devices*—varying from simple one-message buttons to the more complex devices. Among the simpler communication devices are the one-message generating devices. The best-known (but not the only one) is the Bigmack, a device that is programmable and that allows you to repeat the same message over and over again. It can be a great help for beginning communicators, especially individuals who are learning cause-effect relationships. When developing an intervention plan, you can build a learning sequence where the user starts with a single one-message communica-

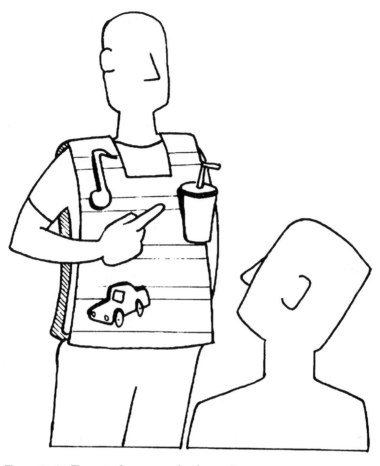

Figure 3–3. The use of a communication vest.

tion device and progresses to two or more one-message devices. This helps users to diversify their responses according to what is appropriate. One can also use multimessage sequential, "step-by-step" devices (where a limited number of messages will be sequentially produced). For example: click 1 will produce "welcome, Keith," click 2 "hang up your coat," and click 3 "go sit in the circle."

At the middle level, there is a whole range of devices that offer the user a limited number of programmable messages, varying from 4 to 128 (Figure 3–4).

Among the more advanced and higher level devices, a distinction is often made between *dedicated* and *nondedicated communication devices*. *Dedicated communication devices* are devices that are built with the sole purpose to be an aid to communication. The *nondedicated devices* have a number of functions and applications that are not limited to communication. In most cases, the nondedicated devices use the platform of laptop or tablet computers with added AAC software.

The distinction between dedicated and nondedicated has some legal significance.

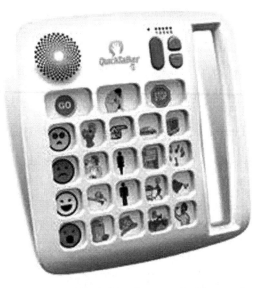

Figure 3–4. The Quicktalker—used with permission from Ablenet.

Insurance companies have long refused to fund a device that they consider to be much more than a prosthesis for speech. They see it as a computer that will allow the user to do much more than just communicating. Personally, I question the wisdom of the insurance companies because it implies that communication would be an isolable function. In reality, the way all individuals function, use language, and communicate reflects a cognitive and linguistic integration. You refer to visual representations when you speak, your thoughts make you think that you have something to say, and it is because you communicate that you feel compelled to structure your thoughts. For an AAC user, it should be considered a major step forward to have a device that integrates and combines both linguistic/communicative and cognitive functions and operations. In a single-subject design study, my former graduate student and assistant Mandy Spear recorded a series of treatment ses-

sions with a client who used an integrated communication device. During half of the time of the sessions, only the speech output program was made available to the client. During the other half, the client could use all the functions of the device. The data showed a significant increase of speech generated output for the periods that the client could pull in pictures, films, texts, and everything that was available on the Internet (Spear, Loncke, & Beck, 2006). It just reminds you that you want to have something to talk about: communication is more likely to work if there is a connection with content (pictures, websites, documents).

Finally, it is important to "personalize" the voice output of the device. Voice quality is considered as a unique feature of a person. Devices usually offer a choice between a set of available male and female voices. Speech scientist Rupal Patel has taken this a step further and creates voice-based recordings that take into account measurements of the vocal tract characteristics of the AAC user (Spiegel, 2013), a very promising development.

Desktop and Laptops

For decades, desktop and laptop computers have been used to run AAC software, often parallel and along with other (non-AAC) applications. Desktop computers have advantages for users with limited mobility, while laptops obviously have more portability.

Tablets and Mobile Devices

Tablets and mobile devices provide a platform that has lowered the threshold to AAC access, for a number of reasons.

They are often relatively inexpensive, have a great portability, are used for multiple daily life functions, and have a high social acceptability. There is no question that the almost sudden rise and omnipresence of iPads and mobile computing has dramatically changed the landscape of AAC, AAC practices, and integration into daily life (Dutton, Scherz, Finch, & Gosnell, 2012). Some believe that this development is much more than merely a technological advancement, but that it changes the nature of AAC in many ways: users appear to choose the tablet platform and start "self-treatment" independently and often prior to seeking advice or input from clinicians or other professionals. For users and others, the many AAC-related apps are often just one of the many tools along apps for articulation, language, phonological, letter recognition, syntax, and more. The use of AAC-related activities tend to become less clinician-driven and more based on the client's choices and decisions (Bradshaw & Bradshaw, 2013; Gosnell, 2011). McNaughton and Light (2013) state: "The iPad and mobile technology revolution has rocketed AAC into the mainstream, offering new options for meeting a breadth of communication needs, increasing public awareness, enhancing adoption by consumers and their families, democratizing access to AAC technologies, and transforming the model of service delivery to one that is clearly consumer driven" (p. 114).

LEXICON-TECHNOLOGY

A lexicon is a database of lexical elements that are organized and stored in some relation to each other. Psycholinguists study the *mental lexicon*, possessed and used by all language users. The mental lexicon is considered to be a highly interconnected and multilayered system of neuropsychological networks. Its organization allows fast access through associative and linguistic (phonological, morphological, syntactic, and semantic) connections—its effective structure allows fast word access (Bonin, 2004). Lexicon-technology tries to emulate the possibilities of speedy access of natural mental lexicons. The mental lexicon can be multimodal (i.e., the lexical items [the words, the manual signs] often have internally stored representations in different codes, e.g., articulatory, visual, acoustic, gestural).

Lexicon Representation

In many AAC applications, the lexicon is represented in a multimodal fashion. For example, graphic symbols are shown along with the printed word and a spoken output possibility. It is assumed that the multimodal representation of symbols allows alternative and mutually reinforcing access routes to the lexical element (e.g., one has the option to recognize the picture or hear and understand the speech output—or both).

However, the most essential characteristic of the lexicon is probably not how the single lexical item is represented, but how the lexical elements are positioned in relation to each other. Is the lexicon structured according to phonological principles (like sound), syntactic principles (word types, e.g., nouns and verbs), semantic networks (with words that belong to the same "theme" positioned together), or simply by frequency? This is important because it probably determines the navigability of the system. The mental lexicon of typical speakers is most likely structured in an "all of the above" way. Speakers use phonological, semantic, frequency, and other associative routes to the lexicon (Paivio, 2010). It is a fast and generally effective process.

Can AAC-technology emulate that? Can AAC devices and software help the user to quickly access a lexical item, and quickly move from there to the next chosen one? One solution that has been offered in AAC is the use of a more limited lexicon that has been carefully selected so that frequently used, "core vocabulary" items are quickly found. The limited number of lexical elements reduces the number of competing lexical items that typically would belong to what is called "fringe vocabulary" (Cannon & Edmond, 2009; see also Chapter 5).

Most of the software used in AAC devices now has word prediction to reduce the number of keystrokes to access the word (and reduce composition and navigation efforts and time). This can be seen as an attempt to accelerate lexical access.

The Super Lexicon and Increasing Interconnectivity

The term "super lexicon" has been proposed by my graduate students in 2012 to indicate a virtual lexicon that contains spoken representations, printed forms, and images of the gesture/manual sign, along with likely "neighboring" lexical items. Technology will likely create a lexicon that is both comprehensive and easily accessible. It will also have an enhanced interconnectivity. "Cloud computing" opens up great possibilities; it allows users to store information (including graphic symbols) that remain available and accessible at different locations and from different devices (Mahmood, 2013).

In the first place, devices are now interconnected and mutually synchronized through Web-Cloud connection. Linked to GPS-technology (Global Positioning Systems), devices can bring up displays and parts of the lexicon that are relevant for the situation. For example, upon entering a restaurant, appropriate phrases ("I believe we have a reservation, my name is Evelyn Flavez") can jump to the foreground within the device.

Growing and Accessible Databases

Using electronic forms of AAC has increasingly implied the possibility of electronically keeping track of all the operations performed by the user. The device can "learn" in which linguistic contexts symbols, words, and phrases are used, and offer the user word and phrase prediction through shortcuts (e.g., fewer keystrokes). The database can be used for other purposes (e.g., keeping track of the linguistic constructions a AAC user has employed that can form a tool for language therapy or, more generally, measurement of communication behavior; see Chapter 11 on assessment). Gomory and Steele (2012) depict a vision of how stored AAC behavior functions can be employed as an input to a cycle that informs clinicians about progress, and that, in turn, can be used for planning intervention (Figure 3–5).

CONVERSION TECHNOLOGY

To comprehend information, it may be required that the symbols (and grammar) used are converted into symbols and systems that can be more easily accessed and interpreted by the user. With the status of

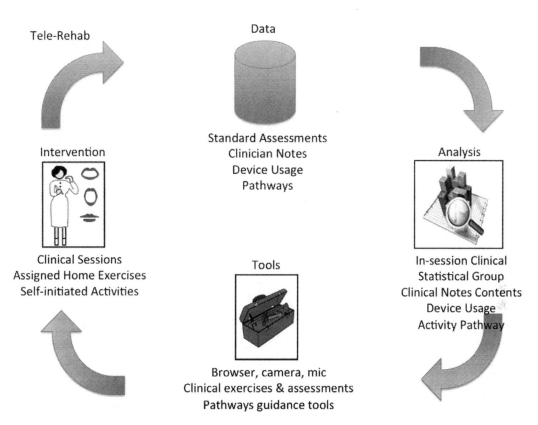

Tele-Rehab

Data

Standard Assessments
Clinician Notes
Device Usage
Pathways

Intervention

Analysis

Clinical Sessions
Assigned Home Exercises
Self-initiated Activities

Tools

In-session Clinical
Statistical Group
Clinical Notes Contents
Device Usage
Activity Pathway

Browser, camera, mic
Clinical exercises & assessments
Pathways guidance tools

Figure 3–5. Electronically and cloud-based data management. © Lingraphica. Used with permission.

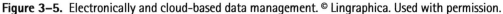

today's technology, the general public has become familiarized with some forms of language translation technology. Examples are *Google translate* (Google, 2013), *Systran* (Systran company, 2013), and *SDL* (Single DirectMedia Layer) Automated translation (SDL, 2013).

Conversion types that are the most relevant for today's AAC are (Ruiter et al., 2012):

- Conversion of spoken language into written language (speech recognition)
- Conversion of written language into spoken language (speech synthesis)

- Modifying written language (summarize, simplify, shorten, paraphrase)
- Conversion of written language into Braille
- Conversion of pictures, pictograms, animations, and sign symbols into speech
- Conversion of text into pictures, graphic symbols, animations, and manual signs.

Word from/to Graphic Symbol

Within AAC, the practice of copresenting graphic symbols with a printed word or phrase has existed since the first years of AAC. Today's commercial graphic symbol software (such as Boardmaker, and others) offers the possibility to convert words to graphic symbols: This is constructed and functions as a search mechanism that links graphic symbols to printed or spoken words.

Manual Sign from/to Word

As mentioned before, at present, software that allows the recognition of manual signs (Jalab, 2012) is under development. Ongoing research includes also a "digital pocket interpreter" (a device that would translate spoken words into signs and vice versa), and conversion technology from a manual signing glove to text (Oz & Leu, 2011).

Simplification Technology

Text simplification can consist of *syntactic simplification* or *lexical simplification*. Syntactic simplification is "the process of reducing the grammatical complexity of a text, while retaining its information content and meaning" (Siddharthan, 2006). Lexical simplification is the use of synonyms or rephrasing formulations in order to make text more accessible to readers (Moropa, 2009).

RECOGNITION TECHNOLOGY

Recognition technology is geared toward interpreting messages that have been expressed as spoken words, as manual signs, or in another form. Within AAC,

this technology is increasingly finding applications as steering technology.

Speech Recognition

(Automatic) Speech recognition is software-based conversion of natural speech into text or another symbolic modality or representation. In its initial years (1980s and 1990s), the technology struggled with difficulties to develop software that would recognize nonstandard speech (e.g., speakers with a foreign accent, or speakers with a speech impairment). In recent years, advances have been made in recognizing lower standard speech such as dysarthric speech (i.e., speech that has a high degree of unintelligibility for unfamiliar listeners) (Selouani, Dahmani, Amami, & Hamam, 2012).

Face Recognition, Gesture, and Sign Recognition

Gesture and manual sign recognition is a field of research that has made enormous progress. Its applications in the field of assistive technology are obvious. The software employed in face and object recognition can be integrated into multimodal networks (Lee et al., 2013).

INTEGRATION WITH OTHER NONCOMMUNICATION TECHNOLOGY

AAC-focused technology has been (and continues to be) applications of technological research and development that is focused on the mainstream public. For example, speech recognition for hand-free steering of instruments and vehicles, and translation software companies have known a commercial success across the world. Also, for AAC users, the technology is not restricted to person-to-person communication, but can also be employed for daily living technology. AAC and other forms of assistive technology can be one integrated personal functional system (Gillette, 2009). For example, persons who rely on eye gaze communication will most likely also use it for turning the television on and off, as well as for writing e-mail messages, surfing the Internet, adjusting their bed position, or other "smart house" functions (Heckman, 2008).

Avatar technology refers to the use of a graphical and often animated character that represents the person. Possibilities to use avatar technology extend from the commercial to the educational sphere (Ang, Bobrowicz, Siriaraya, Trickey, & Winspear, 2013). Within AAC, avatar technology has been employed for animated manual sign language conversions or interpreting. Other possibilities include connecting with others (AAC users or not) in a virtual community.

CONCLUSIONS

In the past few years, technological advances have dramatically changed what is possible in the area of assistive technology in general and particularly in AAC. Devices and solutions that used to be cutting edge solutions (or only in the prototype stage) have become available, miniaturized, more affordable, and more powerful than before. It is to be expected that this evolution will only continue—and that AAC users and

their partners will greatly benefit from this. In order to be able to fully appreciate, apply, and integrate (new as well as more traditional) technology into a person's functioning, it is important to judge where in the communication process the device or the solution is to be situated: is it essentially a word finding (and expression) device? Is it a conversion device? Does it emulate multimodal processing? In the end, these are psycholinguistic processes. Therefore, an evidence-based model of message generation should remain central when one considers the benefits and the effects of a device.

POINTS TO REMEMBER

- Assistive technology involves the use of tools to teach or aid individuals with the goal of allowing them to function more easily in everyday life.
- Assistive technology requires information, training, modeling, counseling, and feedback.
- Recent advancements in technology have allowed AAC devices to become more portable, affordable, and easier to access.
- The advance in mobile computing devices has changed the nature of AAC to become less clinician-directed and more client-directed. Clients more often choose the tablet format and may even start "self-treatment" before seeking advice from clinicians or other professionals.
- Neuroprosthetics is a discipline that seeks to help impairments with motor, sensory, and cognitive functions that uses internal body operations to control the device.

- One-message generating devices may be beneficial for beginning communicators, especially when learning intentional communication (cause-effect relationships). In developing intervention plans, it may be beneficial to start with a simple one-message communication device and then progress to two or more of these devices.
- It is important to keep in mind the level of cognitive functioning of the AAC user when choosing the device, whether it is nontech, low-tech, or high-tech, and also if it is a dedicated or nondedicated device. Some devices have different cognitive levels to facilitate development. Within the type of device, you want to also consider the following regarding the lexicon: multimodal, how they are presented in relation to one another, navigability of the device, core vocal versus fringe vocabulary, and if the device has word prediction technologies. There is a right solution for every person.
- There are many ways to steer/manipulate/direct an AAC device. This includes the following types of input systems: switch-based input system (uses switches or a single switch), pointing based input system (example: mouse, joy-stick, touch screen), audition-based input system (uses voice recognition), and haptic input systems (responds to skin and muscle pressure).
- The terms high-tech and low-tech usually refer to the higher and lower price end of the devices. With the rate at which new technologies continue to become available, at reduced costs, terms like "high" and "low" technology are relative and should be considered on a dynamic continuum.

That is why we should focus more on the functions, components, and processes within communication that can be technologically supported.

REFERENCES

Ang, C. S., Bobrowicz, A., Siriaraya, P., Trickey, J., & Winspear, K. (2013). Effects of gesture-based avatar-mediated communication on brainstorming and negotiation tasks among younger users. *Computers in Human Behavior, 29*(3), 1204–1211.

Assistiveware. (2013). *Proloquo2go*. Retrieved from http://www.assistiveware.com/product/proloquo2go

Bonin, P. (2004). *Mental lexicon: Some words to talk about words*. Hauppauge, NY: Nova Science.

Bradshaw, J., & Bradshaw, J. (2013). The use of augmentative and alternative communication apps for the iPad, iPod and iPhone: An overview of recent developments. *Tizard Learning Disability Review, 18*(1), 31–37.

Bruno, J. (2013). *Gateway to language and learning*. Retrieved from http://www.gatewaytolanguageandlearning.com

Cannon, B., & Edmond, G. (2009). A few good words. *ASHA Leader, 14*(5), 20–23.

Center for AAC and Autism. (2009). *What is LAMP? (language acquisition through motor planning)*. Retrieved from http://www.aacandautism.com/lamp

Cook, A. M., & Hussey, S. M. (1995). *Assistive technologies: Principles and practice*. St. Louis. MO: Mosby.

Dutton, L., Scherz, J., Finch, A., & Gosnell, J. (2012). *iPads and other tablets as AAC devices: Needs, issues, and research*. Workshop at the ISAAC 2012 Research Symposium, Pittsburgh, Pennsylvania (unpublished manuscript).

Fitzgerald, E. (1969; 1949). *Straight language for the deaf; A system of instruction for deaf children*. Washington, DC: Volta Bureau.

Gillette, Y. (2009). Integrating assistive technology with augmentative communication. In G. Soto & C. Zangari (Eds.), *Practically speaking. Language, literacy, and academic development for students with AAC needs* (pp. 265–285). Baltimore, MD: Paul H. Brookes.

Gomory, A., & Steele, R. (2012). Measurement, assessment, and data use cycles in electronically delivered aphasia rehabilitation offerings. *ISAAC Research Symposium,* University of Pittsburgh.

Google, I. (2013). *What is Google translate?* Retrieved from http://translate.google.be/about/

Gosnell, J. (2011). Apps: An emerging tool for SLPs. *ASHA Leader, 16*(12), 10–13.

Hager, E. B. (2012, 07/26; 2013/6). For children who cannot speak, a true voice via technology. *The New York Times,* p. B3(L).

Heckman, D. (2008). *A small world: Smart houses and the dream of the perfect day.* Durham, NC: Duke University Press.

Inman, N. (2013). *WordPower and picture word power.* Retrieved from http://www.inmaninnovations.com

Jalab, H. A. (2012). Static hand gesture recognition for human computer interaction. *Information Technology Journal, 11*(9), 1265–1271.

Just, M. A., & Just, M. A. (1980). A theory of reading: From eye fixations to comprehension. *Psychological Review, 87*(4), 329–354.

Karray, F., Alemzadeh, M., Abou Saleh, J., & Nours Arab, M. (2008). Human-computer interaction: Overview on state of the art. *International Journal on Smart Sensing and Intelligent Systems, 1*(1), 137–159.

Lee, H., Lim, S. Y., Lee, I., Cha, J., Cho, D., & Cho, S. (2013). Multi-modal user interaction method based on gaze tracking and gesture recognition. *Signal Processing: Image Communication; MPEG-V, 28*(2), 114–126.

Mahmood, Z. (2013). *Cloud computing.* Springer-Link ebooks—Computer science. London, UK: Springer-Verlag.

Mayer-Johnson. (2013). *What is Boardmaker?* Retrieved from http://www.mayer-johnson.com/what-is-boardmaker/

McNaughton, D., & Light, J. (2013). The iPad and mobile technology revolution: Benefits and challenges for individuals who require augmentative and alternative communication. *Augmentative and Alternative Communication, 29*(2), 107–116.

Medical Devices. (2004). Stroke patients may regain ability to communicate with speech-enabling device. *Science Letter,* 798.

Moropa, K. (2009). Utilizing "hot words" in Para-Conc to verify lexical simplification strategies in English-xhosa parallel texts. *South African Journal of African Languages, 29*(2), 227–241.

Neuroprosthetics: Fine mind control of machine. (2013). *Nature, 493*(7431), 137.

Oz, C., & Leu, M. C. (2011). American Sign Language word recognition with a sensory glove using artificial neural networks. *Engineering Applications of Artificial Intelligence; Infrastructures and Tools for Multiagent Systems, 24*(7), 1204–1213.

Paivio, A. (2010). Dual coding theory and the mental lexicon. *Mental Lexicon, 5*(2), 205–230.

Quist, R., & Lloyd, L. (1997). Principles and uses of technology. In L. Lloyd, D. Fuller, & H. Arvidson (Eds.), *Augmentative and alternative communication. A handbook of principles and practices* (pp. 197–126). Boston, MA: Allyn & Bacon.

Ricciardi, S., Nappi, M., Paolino, L., Sebillo, M., Vitiello, G., Gigante, G., & Vozella, A. (2010). Dependability issues in visual-haptic interfaces. *Journal of Visual Languages & Computing, 21*(1), 33–40.

Ruiter, M., Beijer, L., Cucchiarini, C., Krahmer, E., Rietveld, T. M., Strik, H., & Hamme, H. (2012). Human language technology and communicative disabilities: Requirements and possibilities for the future. *Language Resources and Evaluation, 46*(1), 143–151.

SDL. (2013). *SDL automated translation.* Retrieved from http://www.sdl.com/products/automated-translation/

Selouani, S., Dahmani, H., Amami, R., & Hamam, H. (2012). Using speech rhythm knowledge to improve dysarthric speech recognition. *International Journal of Speech Technology, 15*(1), 57–64.

Semantic Compaction Systems. *Minspeak.* Retrieved from http://www.minspeak.com/index.php#.UccIFBYudn8

Siddharthan, A. (2006). Syntactic simplification and text cohesion. *Research on Language and Computation, 4*(1), 77–109.

Spear, A., Loncke, F., & Beck, J. (2006). *Effects of multimedia integrated in a speech-generating AAC device* (unpublished manuscript). Poster presented at the Annual Convention of the American Speech-Language and Hearing Association.

Spiegel, A. (2013). *New voices for the voiceless: Synthetic speech gets an upgrade.* NPR radio report.

Steele, R., Aftonomos, L., & Koul, R. (2010). Outcome improvements in persons with chronic global aphasia following the use of a speech-generating device. *Acta Neuropsychologica, 8*(4), 342–359.

Systran Company. (2013). *Systran: The leading supplier of language translation software.* Retrieved from http://www.systransoft.com/systran

Thompson, D., Blain-Moraes, S., & Huggins, J. (2013). Performance assessment in brain-computer interface-based augmentative and alternative communication. *BioMedical Engineering OnLine, 12*(1), 43.

Van Tatenhove, G. (2005). *Language functions and early generative language production* (unpublished manuscript).

Vetulani, Z. (2011). *Human language technology. Challenges for computer science and linguistics* (SpringerLINK Lecture Notes in Computer Science). New York, NY: Springer.

Walkowski, S., Dörner, R., Lievonen, M., & Rosenberg, D. (2011). Using a game controller for relaying deictic gestures in computer-mediated communication. *International Journal of Human-Computer Studies, 69*(6), 362–374.

CHAPTER 4

The Use of Symbols

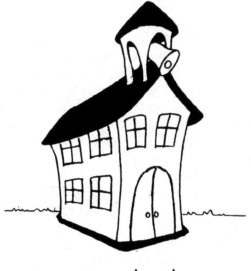

school

WHAT ARE SYMBOLS?

Within AAC, the term "symbols" refers to forms that can be used as communicative behaviors, The symbols represents an idea that the persons wishes to convey. Note that the symbolic value rests solely in the mind of the user: a picture or a manual sign does not have any symbolic meaning unless the user knows or recognizes the meaning (see also Chapter 6).

In the previous chapters, we have already introduced the concept of the use of graphic symbols. We have also mentioned the use of manual signs as an important part of the techniques used in AAC.

In this chapter, we explore these and other "alternative" symbols. The term "alternative" here stands for a modality different than natural speech. In many (maybe most) instances, the "alternative" form is used in some form of combination or configuration together with spoken language. What is "alternative" is not so much the modality itself. After all, almost all of the "alternative forms" are used in typical communication. Everybody uses graphic symbols of some sort in communication, and everybody uses gestures accompanying speech. What is alternative in AAC is that these modalities are brought to the foreground and play a more prominent role.

SYMBOL CLASSIFICATION

Let us first take a look at symbol classification. In the previous chapters, we discussed the difference between *aided* and *unaided* symbols. Briefly stated (Figure 4–1), *unaided symbols* are those that the human body can generate, (i.e. *natural speech, gestures, manual signs,* and *eye blinking codes*). The main advantage of unaided symbols and unaided communication is that you are not dependent on tools. This has its benefits for the naturalness of communication (you carry all your unaided symbols with you all the time), and sometimes the speed of communication. Aided symbols, on the other hand, can pose an "availability problem" (i.e., a dependence on whether the communication board, the device, or another external tool is available and accessible).

Aided symbols include *objects used for communication, graphic symbols,* and a whole range from nontech and low-tech to high-tech *communication devices.* The advantages of the aided symbols can include their *visual nature,* the fact that some symbols are more *static* and have *less variability* (symbols look and sound exactly the same each time you produce them regardless of who produces them), and that they often are easier to access for individuals with limited motor abilities.

One can even talk about the aided-unaided distinction at the level of *symbol selection.* Although unaided symbols can only be selected through an unaided strategy (you can only produce natural speech by speaking; you can only produce gestures by gesturing), aided symbols can be selected through unaided and aided strategies. For example, you can point with your finger (an unaided strategy) to a graphic symbol (an aided symbol), but you can also use a head pointer or a laser pointer (an aided strategy) to activate that same graphic symbol (an aided symbol).

UNAIDED AAC SYMBOLS

Within the category of unaided AAC symbols, a distinction can be made between *nonlinguistic* and *linguistic* symbols. This relates to the question whether the symbols belong to a language, such as an auditory language (a spoken language: English, French, Portuguese, Mandarin,

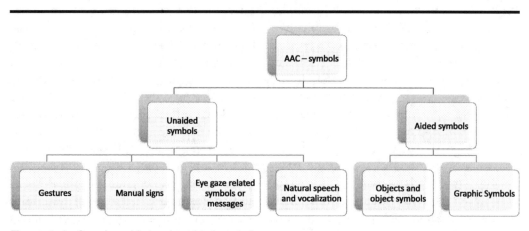

Figure 4–1. Overview aided and unaided symbols.

Swahili, and so on) or a visual language (a signed language: American Sign Language (ASL), Brazilian Sign Language, Chinese Sign Language, South African Sign Language, and others). Among the nonlinguistic unaided symbols, we count different forms of nonlinguistic vocalizations (huh-huh, brrrr, etc.). Most of these are idiosyncratic (i.e., they only have a meaning that is understood by the users themselves and by their partners). A few of these nonlinguistic vocalizations are conventionalized (Ouch!) and understood by a wider community (but don't expect them to have a universally understood meaning).

Yes–No Symbols

As indicated in the previous chapters, it is important to make sure that a person has at least one way of answering *yes-no questions*. This can be done through acoustic symbols (huh-huh being no, and huh-huh with a different intonation contour being yes; again: this is not universal). Of course, yes-no questions can also be answered by using visual nonaided symbols (gestures). The classic yes-no headshake is the most obvious choice. Some clinicians believe we should not even put yes and no symbols on communication boards since most clients have direct, simple, and easily understandable unaided forms of indicating yes and no. Other yes-no answering can include eye-blink codes (i.e., one eye blink is yes, two eye blinks means no—but one can decide on any agreed-upon code).

UNAIDED SYMBOLS: GESTURES

In the past 20 years, major psychological and linguistic research has been con-ducted on *gestures*. Although gestures have been on the radar of psychologists since the beginning of experimental psychology in the 1880s (Wundt, 1973), it is only in the past two decades that we have started to see its importance for cognitive and linguistic processes, as well as for communication disorders in general (and AAC in particular).

Gestures are distinct from manual signs in that they do not belong to a real language system. In a way, many manual signs are gestures that have been "upgraded" into a linguistic organization (aka., a language)—more about that later. Most gestures are a natural by-product of speech (they are produced together with natural speech), whereas manual signs are essentially an equivalent of spoken words. In the sign languages of deaf communities, signs are produced without speech. Adam Kendon (1988), a pioneer in gesture research, has proposed to classify gestures as varying in: (1) linguistic nature, and (2) speech relatedness. Gesture use can be represented on a continuum, which was termed "Kendon's continuum" by McNeill (1992). The continuum shows gesture use from less linguistic to fully linguistic (Figure 4–2). On the left side of the continuum, we see "spontaneous gesticulation": movements and movement patterns of the body with low meaning. These can include what McNeill (1992; Table 4–1) calls the "beats" that one does with the hand and arm, often rhythmically accompanying the words that are spoken, very much like an orchestra conductor using the baton.

As implied above, "beats" and "spontaneous gesticulation" are generally meaningless. They may indicate how much emphasis a person puts on a message. Also, they often tell you how excited the speaker is, but there is usually not a

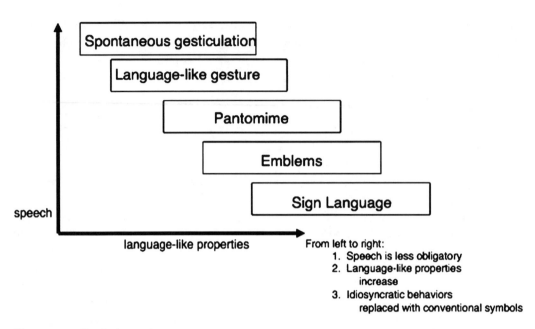

Figure 4–2. Kendon's continuum.

Table 4–1. McNeill's (1992) Gesture Classification

Beats	The hand moves along with the rhythmical pulsation of speech (although the synchrony is not absolutely perfect).
Iconics	A close formal relationship to the semantic content of speech.
Metaphorics	Pictorial-like iconic gestures, but the pictorial content presents an abstract idea.
Cohesives	Can consist of iconic, metaphoric, or pointing gestures, even beats. Gestural cohesion depends on repeating the same gesture form, movement, or locus in the gesture space: the repetition is what signals the continuity.
Deictics	The familiar pointing, or "deictic" gesture.

clear reference to the meaning of a specific unit or idea. Contrary to gesticulation and beats, other types of gestures clearly do carry linguistic characteristics. Here McNeill's classification is helpful (see Table 4–1).

Deictic gestures constitute an interesting subcategory. Deictic gestures are nothing else than pointing in some form —from the typical finger-pointing to pointing with the eyes, with the foot, or whatever is used to indicate the direction of the pointing. Young babies do not point until they are in the second half of their first year of life. It is believed that pointing develops out of grasping and reaching. In early development, pointing is a precursor to labeling and an important avenue to lexical development (Butterworth, 2003). Within AAC, pointing is, for obvious reasons, one of the most powerful access strategies. AAC users point to objects, persons, but also to graphic symbols to express an idea.

Within Kendon's continuum, *"language-like gestures"* are of a different nature. The term means that the gesture is assuming something linguistic. The gesture takes on some value as if it is a word, and often a whole phrase. McNeill makes a distinction between iconic gestures and metaphoric gestures (although both are strongly related to each other). An *iconic* gesture bears some direct resemblance with the physical appearance of the referent. For example, a person might say, "Where is Johnny?" and indicate with the gesture that Johnny is the tall guy (the gesture would mean something like "the tall one"). But if I say, "I have a big idea!" and I spread my arms indicating a wide range from left to right, I am using a *metaphoric* gesture. An idea is an abstract entity, not a concrete object. It is only in our minds that we treat abstract concepts (like ideas) as if they were objects that have measures (big ideas and small ideas). Similarly, if I make a gesture alternately moving my arms up with the hand palms faced up, as if I am weighing something while I say, "I am debating between going to the football game and staying home and getting some work done," I am again using a *metaphoric* gesture. The metaphor is that of scale where I weigh two options as if they were real objects.

The point is that, when people are speaking, they spontaneously generate gestures that are meaningful and that can be exploited—in AAC—as communicative signals. In other words, AAC taps into the potential of individuals to use gestural representations. Psychologists have discovered a number of interesting phenomena about gestures. In the first place, *gestures seem to function as an aid to language processing.* Research shows that individuals gesture more when they have word finding problems—an indication that gesturing helps provide access to their mental lexicon (Krauss, Chen, & Gottesman, 2000). This is one of the reasons why gestures—and manual signs—can be beneficial in AAC, as they may help in accessing and activating the spoken word.

Second, *gesture and speech appear to be two parts of one coordinated action.* In McNeill's theory of gesture and speech, they are two sides of the same coin. Although speech (or spoken language) is more analytical (words and sound are organized/analyzed in a specific serial order), gestures are more imagistic and more global. Interestingly enough, individuals with speech or language disorders inadvertently also display their difficulties in their gestures. Persons, who are disfluent in their speech, are also disfluent in their gesturing (Mayberry, Jaques, & DeDe, 1998). Gesturing by patients with aphasia are sometimes a reflection of their language disorder. Persons with a Broca-type aphasia gesture in a more hesitant, halting, and parsing way, as is their speech. Patients with Wernicke-type aphasia may be much more fluent (Skipper, Goldin-Meadow, Nusbaum, & Small, 2007).

In natural development, gestures appear before speech. Although normal children produce their first spoken words between 10 and 13 months of age, the first gesture comes 2 to 3 months earlier. This is an indication that children are ready for symbolic representations long before they can produce spoken symbols. The reason may be that speech articulation simply requires more fine muscular coordination than gesturing; in fact, speech is one of the most complicated motor actions that humans do. Gestures—and manual signs—are thus an obvious and natural choice to express symbols at a time during development when children are not entirely ready for speech yet. Once normal children acquire sufficient speech articulation skills, spoken language will naturally become the dominant modality of choice. For all children, there is a period in their development when they can express more through gesture than they can through speech. In the 1990s, psychologists Linda Acredolo and Susan Goodwyn (1996) developed a system called *Baby Signs,* which is specially designed for children during this window of development. Baby Signs is a collection of gestures meant for typically developing children. But the rationale behind its introduction and use is very similar to what AAC practitioners try to do: (1) Baby Signs help children to express themselves during periods that speech is developmentally not (yet) available, (2) they do not hinder speech—but, on the contrary, provide a developmental scaffolding that allows natural speech to develop, and (3) they avoid frustration and misunderstanding. Note that this reasoning does not accept the *incompatibility hypothesis.* The incompatibility hypothesis states that different expressive modalities (gesture, speech) are in competition with each other (see Chapter 10). On the contrary, the gesture research and the practical experience with Baby Signs agree on one thing: one should use the most accessible modality (the gesture!) while you wait for

speech to develop. At the same time one counts on the gesture to precisely help the development of speech. These arguments form the rationale of why a collection of gestures can be used as part of a person's repertoire of communication. Because of the *compatibility thesis,* the gestures can be combined with other communication modalities: speech, graphic symbols, and speech-generating devices.

EVERYBODY USES GESTURE

Gestures are a normal phenomenon in the process of development. Everybody uses gestures. Research has shown that even blind children spontaneously develop and use gestures—even if they can hardly benefit from the visual information that is carried by the gesture. It appears that gestures come with internalized psychomotor patterns that help individuals plan their behavior and communication. Gestures are a low-cost and powerful AAC tool, especially for beginning communicators. As an intervention practice, one can observe the idiosyncratic gestures that a child or an adult produces and reinforce these by being consistent in the response (i.e., a basic technique to establish a cause-effect understanding). These behaviors can be considered to be "potential communicative acts" (Sigafoos et al., 2000) if they lead to interpretation and coaching by communication partners (Braddock et al., 2013). It is recommended to initially introduce or reinforce gestures for basic needs and requests (see also Chapter 6). This approach can help the person to establish an initial lexicon that is understood by communication partners. The development of such a personal lexicon can be an important part of an Individualized Education Plan (IEP) or a service or support plan. Figure 4–3 provides an example of how a team of communication partners (e.g., the parents and a teacher) can decide to reward and reinforce gestural behavior in order to "upgrade" it to consistent communicative acts in the repertoire of a person.

As the example in the table shows, a personal and idiosyncratic lexicon can contain directions to follow in terms of how to respond to and encourage the client, including modeling the gestures for communication.

CONVENTIONALIZED GESTURES ARE MANUAL SIGNS

When gestures become conventionalized, even within a community and context of just a few users, they start to function as lexical items. This is the transition from gesture to manual sign. We reserve the term "manual sign" for gestures that are used in a systematic and consistent way in communication. Within AAC, manual signs often are borrowed from an existing sign language (e.g., ASL) but can also be created artificially.

A special system of manual signs or gestures that is not directly derived from a sign language of deaf communities is *Amer-Ind* (Skelly, 1979; Figure 4–4). This

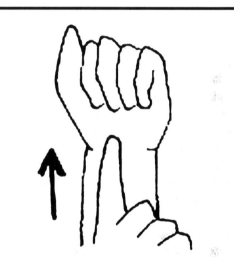

Figure 4–4. Amer-Ind symbol ASCEND.

What John does	What it means	How to respond	Comments
John knocks on the table.	John wants food.	Follow John and interpret.	The gesture will be less idiosyncratic if partners also use gesture.
John takes you by the hand and pulls you toward something.	John wants you to do something.	Follow John and interpret.	This may be an instance to shape and model pointing behavior.
John moves his hand quickly while looking at a drawing pad.	John wants to draw or color.	Give John the drawing pad and comment.	The movement may be shaped toward the WRITE manual sign.

Figure 4–3. Example of a gesture intervention plan.

system is based on the manual communication and signaling system in use by Native Americans up to the 19th century. Skelly discovered that the signs of this system could be helpful in therapeutic communication intervention with individuals with aphasia.

LINGUISTIC UNAIDED SYMBOLS

This brings us to the *linguistic unaided symbols*, an overview of which is given in Table 4–2 (based on Loncke & Bos, 1997). Let's first go back to our classifications. The most common form of linguistic unaided communication is, of course, natural speech—which is not really a form of AAC. However, it should not be forgotten that it is always good practice to accompany most forms of AAC with natural speech.

Let us focus first on manual signing. On the right side of Kendon's continuum, we noticed manual signs and sign language. It is important to explain the difference between these two concepts. Sign language use implies the use of manual signs within a full-fledged language, with its own grammar. These are the languages that have developed in deaf communities: ASL (in the United States), French Sign Language, Korean Sign Language, are just a few examples. It was not until the 1960s and the 1970s that linguists discovered that these languages contained all the same structural complexities as spoken languages. Natural sign languages have a lexicon of thousands of signs, and formational rules (phonology, morphology, and syntax) that regulate how sentences and phrases are formed. The meaning of the term "phonology" for sign languages is to not to be taken literally ("phonology" means "sound system"). It is to be

Table 4–2. Unaided Linguistics Symbol Classification

Category	Type	Examples
Acoustic symbols	Natural speech	Spoken English
Visual symbols	Natural sign languages	American Sign Language
	Artificial sign sets/systems	Gestuno Simplified Sign System
	Manually coded languages	Signed English
	Key word signing	
	Alphabet-based symbols	Fingerspelling/ Morse code
	Phonemic-based symbols	Cued Speech
Tactile symbols	Alphabet-based symbols	Lorm manual alphabet
	Vibrotactile phomenic- or phonic-based symbols	Tadoma

Source: Based on Loncke & Bos, 1997, p. 88.

understood in its structural-linguistic sense: how a set of meaningless elements (the phonemes for a spoken language; for a sign language the hand configurations, the movements, and the locations on or near the body) are assembled and reassembled in different configurations to form meaningful manual signs.

Because sign languages have the same complexity as spoken languages, they do not offer an easy structure. Therefore, sign languages are seldom considered to be a valuable AAC solution. Note that the use of sign language by deaf individuals should not be considered as AAC—it is a natural preference for a language that is expressed and received in the visual-gestural modality, the modality that is intact in deaf individuals (hence the modality that allows deaf individuals to fully develop their linguistic potential). However, *manual signing*—the second concept—is a very powerful and often successful form of AAC intervention for many individuals with a variety of developmental (or other) communication disorders (such as autism spectrum disorders). We are talking here about the practice of systematically teaching individuals to use a limited set of manual signs, often in combination with speech. We should not call this sign language. Within the AAC literature, the term "sign language" is often erroneously used for some coding of spoken language.

A limited set of signs? The reason why manual signing is often limited (sometimes not more than 10 signs) frequently relates to the learning capacity of the individual. The first manual signs that are taught are frequently MORE, NO, STOP, PLEASE, and signs for items that have a high relevance in the person's daily life (MILK, SLEEP, MOMMY,

etc.). This lexicon—the personal repertoire—will typically "grow" as the person expands knowledge, experience, and social networks.

WHY WOULD MANUAL SIGNING WORK?

Why do we expect that some nonspeaking individuals would be able to learn manual signs for communication, when speech is not a viable developmental route? Is manual signing a more accessible option? There are two main reasons to assume that manual signs are easier. The first reason, the *motor argument*, simply states that making manual signs is a motorically easier task than speaking. Remember that speaking is one of the most challenging human neuro-motor coordination activities; it is complex and fast. Manual signs are slower in their production. Even for deaf fluent and native users of sign language, the production of a single sign takes about twice as long as the production of a single word. This does not imply that sign language processing goes more slowly than spoken language processing. Sign languages typically contain more simultaneous information compared with spoken languages, where linguistic information is more often structured sequentially. In spoken language, flexion is often expressed by adding a morpheme (a suffix) to the word (making it longer), whereas sign languages tend to express flexion by modulating the movement pattern or hand configuration of signs (changing the visual outlook, but not making it longer). The relative ease of motor execution is not only related to the fact that it is produced at a slightly lower pace; the neuromuscular patterns are also more on the periphery (the hands and the arms). This latter fact allows people to visually control their own movements and hand configurations. It also makes it possible for an educator or clinician to manually "mold" the fingers, the hands, and the arms of the person—this "molding" technique is sometimes called "hand-over-hand" technique.

The second reason that supports the expectation that some nonspeaking individuals would be able to learn manual signs for communication can be called the *visual argument*. Manual signs are to be processed visually. This visual modality of symbols is thought to be more convenient for many individuals with developmental and communication disabilities who may have limitations with rapid auditory processing. Moreover, the visual modality appears to allow symbols (manual signs and certainly graphic symbols) to have a level of *iconicity*, a degree of resemblance between a symbol and its referent. Iconicity is often rated on a continuum from *transparency* (where the meaning or the referent is obvious for many observers) to *translucency* (where the relation with the referent/meaning first needs to be revealed, before it becomes clear; Lloyd & Blischak, 1992). The ASL sign for CUP is a curved hand (a "C-hand") held with palm orientation to the side on top of a flat hand (a "B-hand") with upward palm orientation. It is easy to "see" the meaning—the sign has a high degree of iconicity. The sign is transparent. The ASL sign SHOE is made with two fist-shape hands, palm facing down, thumbs oriented toward each other, with a movement back and forth toward each other. This sign refers to a part of the motor operation when one is actually tying a shoe. It is not immediately apparent, and not guessable. How-

ever, once it is pointed out, the relation between form and meaning becomes clear. The sign is translucent.

Of course, even for signs with high iconicity, a person needs to have the mental capacity to build and retrieve symbolic internal representations. After all, the symbolic value resides not in the sign itself, but depends on the ability of the user to make the connection with an internal image. Developmental psychology has demonstrated that this is a skill that develops during the first year of life. Piaget called this "the semiotic function" (or symbolic function; Piaget, 1974). It implies that the iconicity of symbols may sometimes not play an important role for individuals who function at a prelinguistic level, who have not reached a level of symbol referential understanding. Interestingly, research shows that young deaf children of deaf parents, who acquire ASL (or another sign language) from very early on, initially ignore the iconic value of the manual signs (Meier, 1991).

Simplified Sign System

Nevertheless, the combination of iconicity and motor ease of manual signs has been shown to be a very powerful AAC technique for many users. In general, developers of signs for AAC use, generally select signs with high iconicity and low motor requirements. This is exactly what psychologist John Bonvillian and his associates have done at the University of Virginia. Bonvillian has developed the Simplified Sign System, a sign communication lexicon designed especially for individuals with severe communicative, developmental, motor, and/or linguistic limitations (Bonvillian et al., 2009). He has put together a lexicon of over 1,000 manual signs for signs/words that are needed for daily communication and are of high frequency use. To do this, Bonvillian selected signs from more than 40 different sources and sign languages, always focusing on signs that would be easy to learn and to execute. He did not base this solely on his intuition; he introduced the selected signs in a series of learning, recognition, and memory experiments involving hundreds of undergraduate students at the University of Virginia. He compared the memory scores of the students for the different manual signs. As a result, the signs that turned out to be the most learnable were the ones that he retained for the Simplified Sign System (Figure 4–5). In his current research and developments, Bonvillian explores the possibility of a simplified sign system for other populations, such as immigrant language learners, and other purposes such as memory training.

How are manual signs used for children and adolescents with AAC needs?

One practice is *key word signing*, a technique of simultaneous communication whereby the communication partner uses natural speech and produces signs for the words that carry the most important information (Windsor & Fristoe, 1991). For example, when saying "please take your coat and hang it up," the caregiver may make the signs for TAKE, COAT, and HANG. This practice is meant to meet several goals. First, it provides multimodality, whereby the communication partner receives linguistic information in two parallel and simultaneous communication modalities. Second, limiting the use of signs to key words reduces the problem of the synchronization between the two channels. This is crucial because producing a sign takes more time than speaking a word—simultaneous production of a signed duplicate of the spoken message would therefore run into the timing problem (Bellugi & Fischer, 1972). Third, it is more conform to the visual nature of signed languages. Signed languages typically do

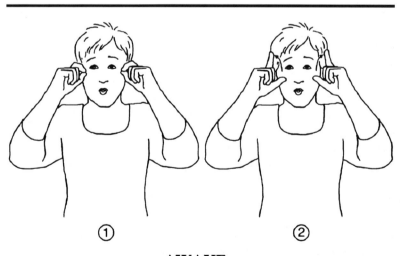

①   ②

AWAKE

Figure 4–5. The simplified sign AWAKE. Courtesy of and permission from John Bonvillian.

not have the same extensive use of "small words" such as prepositions, copulae, and functors. The concepts that lay behind these words (they mainly serve syntactical functions) are expressed in sign languages through modulations of the sign themselves, not through addition of words.

Manual signing is, by definition, a communication method that requires vision. One needs to see the signs. There are, however, sign adaptations possible for hearing impaired individuals with low vision. Hand-over-hand (or tactile) signing is a form of signing where one person signs "on the hands" of the partner. In this form of coactive signing, one person holds the hands of the other while signing together. This form of communication requires an ability to subtly perceive and indicate which movements one wishes to make. In co-active forms of communication, it is sometimes hard to make a clear distinction between sender and receiver—or, to put it differently, to determine who is the actual "author" of the message. This is an issue that has been raised in relation to *facilitated communication*, a technique in which the communication partner holds the hand or arm of the communicator while messages are expressed or interpreted. It is not always clear who is "leading" or "initiating," and how much interpreting there is (Jacobson, Mulick, & Schwartz, 1995). The blurred distinction between sender and receiver has, to this day, made Facilitated Communication a highly controversial technique.

The use of *manual signing* is presently a widespread approach, often in combination with other forms of AAC. However, manual signing is certainly not the only form of linguistic unaided AAC. The use of the *manual alphabet* and all its derivative forms is also a potentially powerful means of alternative linguistic communication. Contrary to most forms of manual signing that use signs borrowed from the natural sign languages of deaf communities, the manual alphabet refers to orthography—which, in turn, is based on spoken language (not sign language). The use of the manual alphabet is often called *fingerspelling*. The advantage of fingerspelling is that it offers a specific and accurate means to convey messages. Historically, this was the approach of the so-called *Rochester method* for deaf children (Marschark, Sapere, Convertino, & Pelz, 2008). The disadvantage is that it requires excellent literacy skills, fine motor skills, and exceptional skills to "read" fast moving and changing successive hand configurations. The manual alphabet is essentially a transmission of the letters of the alphabet into hand shapes, sometimes referred to as "writing in the air."

Even though fingerspelling requires exceptional rapid visual processing skills, there are, however, adaptations of the alphabet-principle for deaf individuals with low vision. Just as hand-over-hand signing and coactive signing introduced a tactile element in the communication, the Lorm alphabet (named after Hieronymus Lorm (1820–1902), the developer of the system) is interactive, and uses touching specific areas on the hand palm of the communication partner (Figure 4–6). Different spots on the hand palm represent the letters of the alphabet. The communication partner "types" the message by touching the projected spots on the hand palm. This skill requires both a strongly internalized representation of the positions on the hand palm as well as excellent literacy skills. Finally, the Tadoma method (Reed, Durlach, Braida, & Schultz, 1989) is based on the learned ability of individuals

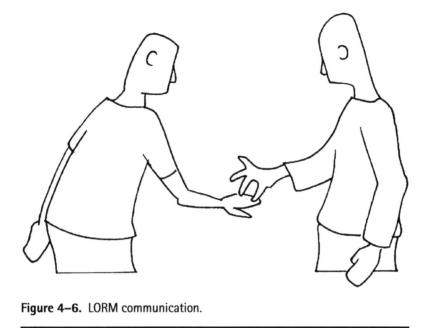

Figure 4–6. LORM communication.

to perceive articulatory patterns by touching the lips, the chin, and the jaw of the person. This method is rarely used but interesting—it is a tactile form (or rather a vibrotactile form) of lipreading (or speechreading) for deaf-blind individuals. The deaf-blind listener places a thumb on the lips of the speaker while holding the fingers on the region of the throat and jaw. By doing so, the listener receives tactile information of the ongoing speech articulation process (vocal fold vibration indicating voiceness, jaw opening giving cues about formants, and the movements that convey information about transition between articulemes).

AIDED AAC SYMBOLS

Many forms of aided communication in AAC entail some use of visual informa-

tion. Since the earliest days of AAC, picture communication or, more generally, graphic symbols have been used.

GRAPHIC SYMBOLS

Among the aided communication symbols, the most used and well-known are certainly different forms of graphic symbols. There are a wide variety of graphic symbol systems (and sets). Why is it so commonly in use, and why is it expected by so many to be so powerful? Let us first focus on the rationale why graphic symbols are being used so widely with individuals with AAC needs. There are five reasons:

1. *Graphic symbols are presented in the visual modality*—As indicated, there is reason to believe that many individuals

with developmental and communication disorders have a preference for information processing in the visual modality.

2. *Graphic symbols can be combined with speech*—This allows for multimodality with symbol use in two parallel simultaneous channels (speech and graphic symbols). Generally, it is recommended that caregivers and communication partners speak and comment while the person points to (or indicates otherwise) the graphic symbols. Graphic symbols are often displayed on buttons in speech-generating communication devices—linking the graphic symbol with device-generated speech.

3. *Graphic symbols are static and invariant*—Contrary to the speech signal (which is highly variable and different each time it is produced), graphic symbols retain the same physical visual appearance each time you look at them. It does not require the rapid processing that speech requires (because the acoustic signal is dynamic).

4. *Graphic symbols contain references to the physical and visual world*—Even more than is the case with manual signs, graphic symbols can have strong iconic value (one would almost say that this is so by definition: "iconic" means nothing else than "picture-like"). However, the iconic nature of graphic symbols can be somewhat deceiving. Because a spoken or written word can have many referents (the word "house" refers to a building that can look very different—it can also refer to abstract notions like "the house of Windsor") by choosing a specific picture (a typical dwelling, for example), one runs the risk to be "locked in" to a specific type of refer-

ent (and make the symbol unusable or at least more problematic for other meanings).

5. *Graphic symbols are less abstract than words*—The symbols invite the observer to create an internal picture. Even when the concept to be pictured is abstract, the graphic artist must come up with a visualized concept.

However, in order to be able to capitalize on the potential of graphic symbols, the user must have well-developed internal visual representational skills. Although for adults and most children older than five (and most adults) a picture is usually an easily understandable reference to the outside world, it requires a certain level of development. Psychologists (e.g., DeLoache, 2011) have tried to identify how infants and babies gradually develop these "picture understanding skills." Their research shows that we should not take for granted that individuals with severe developmental delays (even adults) will have the ability to "understand" and immediately grasp (and thus be helped by) the picture and its referent.

Graphic symbol understanding is a "dual representational act," the symbol is an object in itself and it is at the same time a reference to something else. If you say "that is a tiny picture of a huge castle," you comment on the picture (tiny) as well as on the referent (huge castle). During initial development, infants and babies only treat graphic symbols as objects, not as referents. It takes typically developing children up to the age of 18 months before they start to grasp that pictures have conventional referential value. Young children may not be bothered by the fact that you hold a picture upside down. Full pictorial competence can take several years to fully develop. Therefore, educators should not assume a developed pictorial ability for users who are in early developmental stages.

LEVELS OF UNDERSTANDABILITY OF GRAPHIC SYMBOLS

When talking about AAC graphic symbols, it may be helpful to distinguish degrees of learnability and abstractness, and classify gestures into: (1) Recognizable graphic symbols, (2) Guessable graphic symbols, and (3) Symbols with low picturability.

Recognizable Graphic Symbols

These are symbols that refer to concrete referents that often are part of the environment or culture. The symbols have a high transparency, which means that members of the same culture are likely to interpret the symbols in a similar way. Most likely, the interpretation can be captured in a noun. Figure 4–7 shows a few of recognizable graphic symbols.

In our lab observations, all the participants without exception and regardless of their cultural or national background, recognized the symbols in Figure 4–7

as "baby—scissors—key." Why are the graphic symbols in Figure 4–7 highly recognizable? Obviously, they have a high transparency and have no conceptual competitors (there are no other interpretations). Our lab participants had to think hard to come up with "alternative names" (in response to the question "can you think of another name of these?"). As long as the users are familiar with things and customs of the culture and environment, they should "know" what they mean. Common sense dictates that it is preferable to use symbols that have this high-level of transparency.

The fact that there may not be many conceptual competitors is probably not the only reason why a symbol is easily recognized. The way the referent is represented matters too. Most children will recognize a picture of a cat, and our intuition suggests that it doesn't seem to matter much which picture you use: a black and white picture of a cat, a color picture, a more stylized representation. A cat is a cat. Is that really the case? Not quite! Semanticists explain that some cats are "more cat" than others! The degree of "catness" is related to the number of typical cat-features there are, and at the same time to the absence of distracting nonrelevant features.

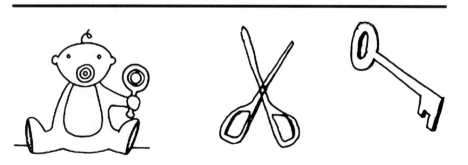

Figure 4–7. Recognizable graphic symbols.

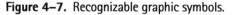

Let's look at these two pictures of a bicycle (Figure 4–8).

These two pictures have been used in our lab in a series of try outs to identify the most recognizable items. Most of the lab participants agreed that both would be fine and easy to recognize, but there is a slight preference for the bicycle on the right. Why? Many participants expressed the opinion that the cartoon-type bicycle on the left may cause some hesitation because it is less "prototypical." Semanticists have indeed suggested that language users store information around prototypes—members of categories that carry the essential and salient features. This explains why every single participant in our lab rejects the bicycle shown in Figure 4–9 (a photograph taken at the Bicycle Museum in Nijmegen, the Netherlands).

Why not you might ask? When exploring the reasons why my students

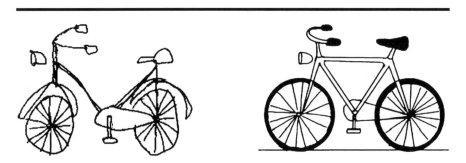

Figure 4–8. Bicycle pictures: Which one is better?

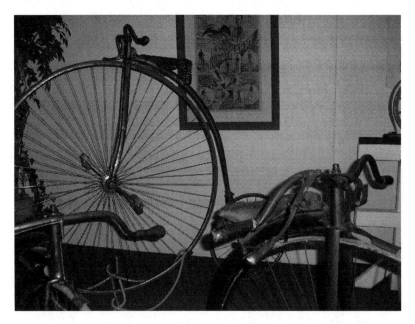

Figure 4–9. A bicycle from the Nijmegen (the Netherlands) bicycle museum.

intuitively but unanimously rejected this picture, we easily came to the conclusion that a good graphic symbol should: (1) contain the most salient characteristics of the object—but not too many more as it might become distractive, (2) allow for "universal" interpretation—observers need to tend to agree what they are seeing, and (3) be detached of a distractive background or additional elements. The picture of the 19th-century bicycles violates all these principles. The museum bicycle does not have the typical characteristics—it is not a prototype that we think of as bicycles. The picture may not be universally recognized (you need to have some historical-cultural knowledge and background to know that these are bicycles), and there is distracting background.

Semantic Prototypes

We are thus in search of semantic prototypes (i.e., the representations that individuals feel have the "right relationship between form and meaning"). Rosch (1975) describes a prototype as a relatively abstract mental representation that assembles the key attributes or features that best represent instances of a given category (Evans & Green, 2006, p. 249). Prototypes are culturally sensitive. For example, when I showed a series of cups to both my American and European students (separately), asking which one represents the more prototypical cup (Figure 4–10), the American and European students consistently showed different preferences (but they all rejected the sports cup).

All of this shows that in general, we often do not favor the use of photographs —precisely because photographs may contain so much information. Drawings, on the other hand, can focus on the essence of the thing that is represented. Photographs are nevertheless ideal when we are not representing a category or prototype, but a specific representative, person, or item (the client's mom, pet, room, etc.).

Guessable Graphic Symbols

Graphic symbols can be situated on a transparency—translucency continuum. Guessable symbols are closer to the translucency side of the continuum. These are symbols whose relation to the meaning becomes apparent once the meaning is revealed (Figure 4–11). In these cases, the relation between the picture and the meaning needs to be established through

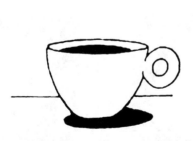

Figure 4–10. Cups and prototypes.

teaching. Educators and clinicians sometimes tend to underestimate this problem because pictures are often accompanied with a caption, a "translation" of the pictures, which makes guessing the meaning easy for individuals who can read. Again, we can illustrate this by comparing a communication board with a copy where the captions have been made illegible—much like a nonliterate person perceives them.

SYMBOLS WITH LOW PICTURABILITY

Low picturability symbols are those in which the iconicity and guessability degree is limited (Figure 4–12). Most of the words in English (and any language) are abstract or pose problems when one attempts to represent them with a graphic symbol. This is the case with all the verbs. For example, take the word "jump." How will you represent "jump"? One usually uses cartoon-like conventions like arrows and circles, describing the pathway of the movement. What you see on the picture is not "jump" but a person in a position before, during, or after the action of jumping—the artist has to use a different set of graphic codes to tell you something about the activity (the pathway and the direction of the jump are in the arrow). Reading this type of cartoon-like graphical symbols requires a developmental level of at least 5 or 6 years, combined with a familiarity with the culture of cartoon conventions.

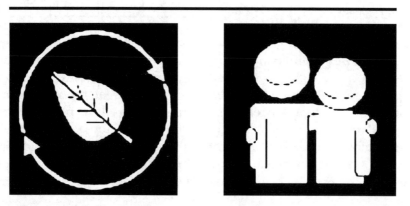

Figure 4–11. Guessable graphic symbols (autumn, friend). Reproduced with permission from http://www.sclera.be/en/vzw/home.

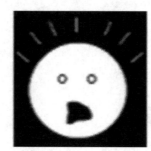

Figure 4–12. Low picturability graphic symbols (first, startled, bad). Reproduced with permission from http://www.sclera.be/en/vzw/home.

AN INTERESTING GRAPHIC SYMBOL SYSTEM: BLISS-WORDS

A graphic communication system that has been used by many AAC users across the world is *Bliss-words*, formerly named *Blissymbolics*. This system is based on the "Semantography" lexicon, developed and published by Charles Bliss in 1949 and in 1965. Bliss was born into a Jewish family in the Austro-Hungarian empire in 1897. As a young man he lived through the difficult periods of World War I, the interwar years, and World War II. After the Nazis took over Austria in 1938, he was interned in a concentration camp. The fact that he was married to a Catholic woman saved his life. He was able to leave Europe, go to Shanghai and, after the war to Australia, where he spent the rest of his life until his death in 1985. He was convinced that war and human suffering find some of their causes in unsuccessful communication. His life experience had a strong influence on his motivation to find a communication system that would bring people together in peace.

Bliss was intrigued by the possibilities of building a "logical" graphic symbol system that should be easy to learn and that would make it possible to avoid miscommunications between people. He considered his work to be a contribution to the improvement of world communication and, indirectly, to world peace. His work initially attracted minimal interest and more skepticism than enthusiasm from linguists or scholars in semiotics. In fact, he was largely considered to be an eccentric and was not taken too seriously by academicians. In the early 1970s, Shirley McNaughton, a special educator at the Ontario Crippled Children's Centre (now the Bloorview MacMillan Centre) in Toronto discovered the system and recognized the possibilities for AAC. She started to use it as a communication system for nonspeaking children with cerebral palsy. Many of her students had normal intellectual capacities and needed a system to express their thoughts and messages. The system became popular and was introduced to many children and adolescents around the world, especially in Canada, the United Kingdom, the Netherlands, France, Australia, and the Scandinavian countries (Bliss & McNaughton, 1976). Bliss-words is probably one of the most "language-like" graphic symbol systems. A natural language uses a limited number of phonemes (English has, depending on who counts and how, between 35 and 42 phonemes; other languages have similar numbers) that are combined to form thousands of different words. Bliss-words uses a similar principle—a "logical principle" as Bliss called it himself: a limited number of graphic forms (somewhat comparable with phonemes or morphemes) are combined and recombined in the symbols. For example, the symbols for "house" and "feeling" combine into the symbol "home." Morphological markers (called indicators) are used to distinguish singular from plural, verbs from nouns, and concrete from abstract symbols. As such, Bliss-words appeals to a person's morphological capacity to create, recognize, and mentally store combinations of a discreet number of elements to form meanings. Symbols are compounds of elements that each form part of the meaning (e.g., "surgeon" is a combination of "person," "medical," and "knife"). The same elements are used to form numerous other words.

The similarity with the structure of natural languages is obvious: just as in a natural language, Bliss has a sublexical level (elements of a system that are combined to form lexical elements; Figure 4–13), and there are rules to combine. There are morphological classifiers, such as a symbol for "four-legged animals."

Reportedly, children and adults learn and use the system in a creative and generative way. For example, they use a marker "opposite" in ways that are similar to the use of the English suffix "un-."

The use of such a system possibly appeals to a person's internal linguistic skills—maybe more than the other graphic symbols systems do (McNaugh-

ton, 1998). There have been a number of studies that look into the question whether the formational characteristics of Bliss-words (the fact that they can be broken down into "sublexical" elements) has an effect on learnability (Carmeli & Shen, 1998; Rajaram, Alant, & Dada, 2012; Shepherd & Haaf, 1995). Proponents of the system emphasize that its value is more than that of a collection of "pictures," but that if offers a system that facilitates mental storage, lexical access, metalinguistic skills, and transition to literacy (Jennische, 2012).

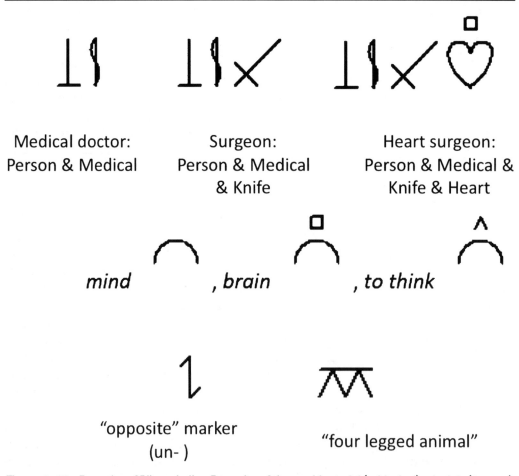

Figure 4–13. Examples of Blissymbolics: Examples of the combinatorial (sublexical) principle (*top row*), the use of qualifiers (*middle row*), and markers and classifiers (*bottom row*). Reproduced with permission.

TWO ISSUES OF GRAPHIC SYMBOLS: POLYSEMY AND SEQUENTIALITY

There are many clinical and educational applications of graphic symbols. Besides the use of symbols on communication boards and displays, as exchange pictures, and on schedules, graphic symbols are also used in storybooks, or as part of language therapy (sentence building activities).

The Polysemy Issue

Polysemy stands for "multiple meanings." It is a term from linguistic semantics that refers to the fact that words have multiple meanings. When you look up the word "line" in the Webster Dictionary, you realize that it is both a verb and a noun. The verb has four meanings (somewhat related, but still different), and the noun has more than 20. "Line" is not exceptional at all. On the contrary, words with a single meaning are the hardest to find. This helps us realize the problem that arises when you select a graphic symbol and put an English word under it. Which meaning do we select for the picture? And do we expect the user to be able to generalize the picture to all meanings of the word?

For example, you might select a picture of a person falling for "fall" (again, the problem with verbs is that you cannot really put them in a picture). You may decide to draw a picture of a person and indicate through the person's body posture and with arrows, facial expression, that he or she is about to fall. But will you also use this picture for the fall season or to construct a sentence with "falling in love"? Here we see that the iconic charac-teristics of the graphic symbols (the physical resemblance) can at the same time be a blessing (easier to learn), and a curse (you are locked into one meaning) at the same time!

It is important to realize that graphic symbols and words cannot be full substitutes for each other. When one thinks of "the graphic symbol for _____ (fill in a word)," one easily falls in the trap of the intuitive (but wrong) assumption that there is a one word—one meaning—one graphic symbol relation. However, there is little agreement—or little discussion—about the question if the symbol stands for all the meanings of the English word or not. If it is supposed to stand for all the meanings, than it really requires an enormous effort of abstract thinking (i.e., not being fooled or distracted by the physical appearance of the symbol). The physical appearance—the initial iconicity—makes it harder to activate the meaning. Ironically, in AAC practice, we selected iconic symbols in the first place to make it easier to learn, not harder!

The Sequentiality Issue

This problem is even more apparent if you want to use graphic symbols in a sequence to express messages composed of several symbols. Several symbol systems allow the user to combine them in a series of ways similar to a spoken or a written language. However, the pictorial characteristics of the graphic symbols make these combinations strange. Take a look at the graphic symbols in Figure 4–14.

These symbols could have been the symbols for "horse" and "run." Earlier, we described the problem of low picturability symbols, and we indicated that, in fact, all verbs had a low picturability.

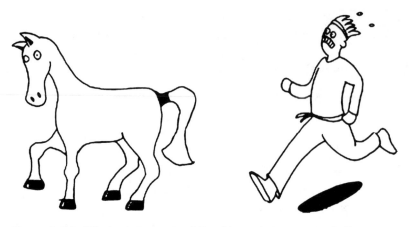

Figure 4–14. "The horse is running." Graphic symbol sequence challenges.

If you want to read the sequence in Figure 4–14 as "the horse runs," you need to make abstraction of the pictorial qualities of the second symbol. By doing this, we are forced to move away from one of the very reasons why many practitioners believed we should use graphic symbols in the first place (i.e., the iconicity). Or, to put it differently, the iconicity is putting the reader on the wrong track here.

USES FOR GRAPHIC SYMBOLS

As discussed previously, graphic symbols are used in different ways as communication tools. We use graphic symbols on communication boards, schedules, as labels on objects, in picture-exchange systems, and certainly on speech generating communication devices.

With today's software, it has become easy to quickly produce *communication boards* and *communication displays* (for communication devices).

When you make a communication board for a person, it is good to remember a few rules and principles that will better the chances of contributing to the person's quality of life.

1. The use of any communication device depends on learning and familiarization (one does not learn to use anything on the first try) by the users as well as by their partners.
2. A learning process needs to be planned starting with a limited number of graphic symbols—to be used in highly motivating and transparent situations.
3. The number of graphic symbols on a communication board should depend on: (a) memory capacity (knowing where the symbols are) and (b) perception and motor abilities (able to see and physically point to or activate the graphic symbols).
4. One needs to consider whether the communication board is a stand-alone board (to be used in multiple situations), a situation-specific board (for the clinic, for the classroom, for a specific activity), or a board that is available to the user along with other boards or displays (e.g., pages in a binder, screens to navigate through).

5. If multiple boards or screens are available, one must be aware that navigation may be a challenge (know where to find the symbols and how to get there) and threatened by time pressure (remember that AAC users often do not even come close to a "normal" rate of conversation). It may, therefore, be a good idea to have some of the most important (the most needed, the most used) graphic symbols repeated on each screen in the same location.

6. For users who are literate, it is a good idea to provide a letter board. The alphabet is the best example of a system that allows you to say anything with a limited number of symbols (the letters of the alphabet, and a space bar and delete key or backspace).

7. One might think of having yes, no, stop as symbols on each board. As discussed before, if the users and their communication partners have developed good interactive strategies, they can basically talk about anything just with the yes-no strategy. Some clinicians and educators object to using board space for yes and no, especially if the users have developed other nonverbal techniques such as head nodding, or eye blinking. Nevertheless, having the symbols on the board makes it more likely that miscommunications will be avoided.

8. As for any communication intervention tool, quality of life, safety, and protection of the individual, are important considerations. STOP and NO are just little things that can help a person to express rejection. Sadly enough, individuals with limited communication are among the most vulnerable for a whole range of abuses (including neglect, verbal abuse, financial abuse, physical abuse, and sexual abuse). Obviously, the vulnerability is related to the inability to verbally fight back and/or to report. Educators, clinicians, and counselors need to be aware of this problem. Placing NO and STOP on a communication board will not prevent much, but it may be part of an awareness education toward users to help them to understand that specific behaviors are wrong and how to respond to them.

9. Is there an emergency plan? You might consider including messages like, "help!," "please call my mom at 123-456-7890," and "I need my medication, it is in the bag behind my wheelchair."

10. Initially, the focus can be on providing the user with messages that will help with their needs and wants ("I need to use the bathroom," "I am hungry," "I want some more"), but one should also think of the need to socialize. You may want to include messages that help the users to introduce themselves ("My name is Gerald. Please be patient, I use this card"), and for small talk, "how are you?"

At the end of the day, the effectiveness of the communication board will depend on many factors. There is not one "right" type of communication board. Users, educators, and clinicians will always need to strike a balance between having a multitude of messages/symbols available (which increases the likelihood of good quality of conversation) and the ease with which it will be operated (more messages to choose from and more navigation will decrease the speech of communication).

In fact, there are many things we don't know or understand yet about communicating with a communication board.

What will work best? Should you spatially group all the nouns together and all the verbs together? Should you organize the symbols by topic? How many symbols would be too much? There has been little research into these questions.

Traditionally, the communication boards (and screens) used to have the "grid" layout, in which symbols and messages are organized in rows and columns. Is that the most intuitive way of organizing a lexicon? That is probably not the case for young children. Individuals with mental challenges or older persons struggling with mental deterioration may sim-

ply find it too hard to grasp. In the past decade, developers have used the touchscreen technology to develop computer *visual scene displays* (Dietz, McKelvey, & Beukelman, 2006). Instead of using the grid-structure, the screen can present anything (a picture, a photograph, or a combination of any visual information). The screen has hidden "hot spots," activation of which will bring up a new screen or deliver a spoken message (Figure 4–15).

The use of visual scene displays has recently attracted attention and triggered research into its possibilities. Visual Scene Displays are generally considered to be an

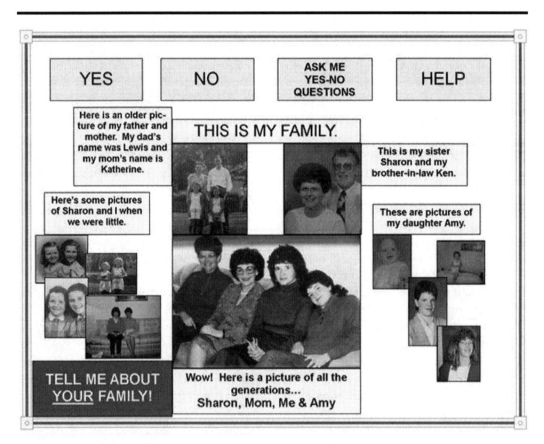

Figure 4–15. Example of visual scene displays. Provided by Dr. Linda Meyer, Woodrow Wilson Rehabilitation Center. Fishersville, VA.

important step in the direction of making AAC devices and methods more intuitive and more accessible.

CONCLUSIONS

The use of nonstandard modalities as an alternative or as an augmentation of standard forms of communication is probably the most essential characteristic of AAC. Understanding the nature of these AAC symbols, aided or unaided, helps us to grasp the reasons why AAC could work.

POINTS TO REMEMBER

- Symbolic value rests only in the mind of the user, the picture, or manual sign has no symbolic meaning unless the user knows or recognizes the meaning.
- When gestures become conventionalized, even if it is just among a small community or group of users, they begin to function as lexical items. This is how gestures transition to manual signs.
- Kendon's Continuum relates to the linguistic meaning behind a gesture. On the low end, we see automatic body movements (unstructured body language), and on the high-end there is sign language (includes sign systems such as ASL).
- Gestures seem to function as an aid to language processing. This is why we suggest utilizing gesture as a therapeutic technique for word finding problems, as well as access stimulation for AAC users. Also,

disfluent gestures can be indicative of disfluent speech.
- Bliss words may lack iconicity, but as a system, it encourages linguistic cognitive skills needed for growth and development ("mental storage, lexical access, metalinguistic skills, and transition to literacy").
- When making a communication board for an individual, it is important to remember to include ways for them to communicate their wants and needs as well as ways for them to protect themselves and socialize with others.
- Implementing a communication device is a "learning process" for both the user and the communication.
- Key word signing can be used as a technique for children and adolescents with AAC needs (in term of using manual signs). Key word signing is when the communication partner of the individual with AAC needs, uses both signs and natural speech simultaneously (the user receives linguistic information in two modalities).

REFERENCES

Acredolo, L. P., & Goodwyn, S. W. (1996). *Baby signs: How to talk with your baby before your baby can talk.* Chicago, IL: Contemporary Books.

Bellugi, U., & Fischer, S. (1972). A comparison of sign language and spoken language. *Cognition, 1*(2), 173–200.

Bliss, C. K., & McNaughton, S. (1976). *The book to the film Mr. Symbol Man.* Sydney, Australia: Semantography-Blissymbolics.

Bonvillian, J. D., Dooley, T., Emmons, H., Jack, A., Kissane, N., & Loncke, F. (2009). *The development of a simplified manual sign communication system for special populations.* 2008 Clinical AAC Research Conference. Charlottesville, VA.

Braddock, B., Pickett, C., Ezzelgot, J., Sheth, S., Korte-Stroff, E., Loncke, F., & Block, L. (2013). Potential communicative acts in children with autism spectrum disorders. *Developmental Neurorehabilitation.* Advance online publication.

Butterworth, G. (2003). Pointing is the royal road to language for babies. *Pointing: Where language, culture, and cognition meet* (pp. 9–33). Mahwah, NJ: Lawrence Erlbaum Associates.

Carmeli, S., & Shen, Y. (1998). Semantic transparency and translucency in compound Blissymbols. *AAC: Augmentative and Alternative Communication, 14*(3), 171–183.

DeLoache, J. S. (2011). Early development of the understanding and use of symbolic artifacts. *The Wiley-Blackwell handbook of childhood cognitive development* (2nd ed., pp. 312–336). New York, NY: Wiley-Blackwell.

Dietz, A., McKelvey, M., & Beukelman, D. R. (2006). Visual scene displays (VSD): New AAC interfaces for persons with aphasia. *Perspectives on Augmentative and Alternative Communication, 15*(1), 13–17.

Evans, V., & Green, M. (2006). *Cognitive linguistics: An introduction.* Mahwah, NJ: Lawrence Erlbaum Associates.

Jacobson, J. W., Mulick, J. A., & Schwartz, A. A. (1995). A history of facilitated communication: Science, pseudoscience, and antiscience science working group on facilitated communication. *American Psychologist, 50*(9), 750–765.

Jennische, M. (2012). *Characteristics of blissymbolics.* Presentation at the International Society for augmentative and alternative communication research seminar. Pittsburgh, PA.

Kendon, A. (1988). How gestures can become like words. In F. Potyatos (Ed.), *Crosscultural perspectives in nonverbal communication* (pp. 131–141). Toronto, Canada: Hogrefe.

Krauss, R., Chen, Y., & Gottesman, R. (2000). Lexical gestures and lexical access: A process model. In D. McNeill (Ed.), *Language and gesture* (pp. 261–283). New York, NY: Cambridge University Press.

Lloyd, L., & Blischak, D. (1992). AAC terminology policy and issues update. *Augmentative & Alternative Communication, 8*(2), 104–109.

Loncke, F., & Bos, H. (1997). Unaided AAC symbols. In L. Lloyd, D. Fuller, & H. Arvidson (Eds.), *Augmentative and alternative communication. A handbook of principles and practices* (pp. 80–106). Boston, MA: Allyn & Bacon.

Marschark, M., Sapere, P., Convertino, C., & Pelz, J. (2008). Learning via direct and mediated instruction by deaf students. *Journal of Deaf Studies and Deaf Education, 13*(4), 546–561.

Mayberry, R., Jaques, J., & DeDe, G. (1998). What stuttering reveals about the development of the gesture-speech relationship. *New Directions for Child Development, 79*, 77–87.

McNaughton, S. (1998). *Reading acquisition of adults with severe congenital speech and physical impairments: Theoretical infrastructure, empirical investigation, educational application.* (Unpublished doctoral dissertation). University of Toronto, Toronto, Canada.

McNeill, D. (1992). *Hand and mind: What gestures reveal about thought.* Chicago, IL: University of Chicago Press.

Meier, R. P. (1991). Language acquisition by deaf children. *American Scientist, 79*(1), 60.

Piaget, J. (1974 [1926]). *The language and thought of the child.* New York, NY: New American Library. [Le langage et la pensée chez l'enfant (M. Gabain, trans.). Delachaux et Niestle. Neuchatel, Switzerland].

Rajaram, P., Alant, E., & Dada, S. (2012). Application of the self-generation effect to the learning of Blissymbols by persons presenting with a severe aphasia. *AAC: Augmentative and Alternative Communication, 28*(2), 64–73 (38 ref).

Reed, C. M., Durlach, N. I., Braida, L. D., & Schultz, M. C. (1989). Analytic study of the Tadoma method: Effects of hand position on segmental speech perception. *Journal of Speech and Hearing Research, 32*(4), 921–929.

Rosch, E. (1975). Cognitive representations of semantic categories. *Journal of Experimental Psychology: General, 104*(3), 192–233.

Shepherd, T. A., & Haaf, R. G. (1995). Comparison of two training methods in the learning and generalization of Blissymbolics. *AAC: Augmentative and Alternative Communication, 11*(3), 154–164 (21 ref).

Sigafoos, J., Woodyatt, G., Deen, D., Tait, K., Tucker, M., Roberts-Pennell, D., & Pittendreigh, N. (2000). Identifying potential communicative acts in children with developmental and physical disabilities. *Communication Disorders Quarterly, 21*, 77–86.

Skelly, M. (1979). *Amer-ind gestural code based on universal American Indian talk.* Amsterdam, Netherlands: Elsevier/North Holland.

Skipper, J. I., Goldin-Meadow, S., Nusbaum, H. C., & Small, S. L. (2007). Speech-associated gestures, Broca's area, and the human mirror system. *Brain and Language; Gesture, Brain, and Language, 101*(3), 260–277.

Windsor, J., & Fristoe, M. (1991). Key word signing: Perceived and acoustic differences between signed and spoken narratives. *Journal of Speech and Hearing Research, 34*(2), 260–268.

Wundt, W. (1973 [1921]). *The language of gesture* (J. S. Thayer, C. M.Greenleaf, & M. D. Silverman, trans.). The Hague, Netherlands: Mouton.

CHAPTER 5

Vocabulary and AAC

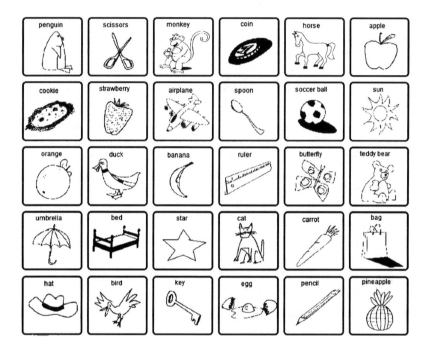

Words are like the bricks of the building called "language." The words (the lexical elements) that a person possesses are stored in a mental lexicon. Some words are typically acquired at a very young age and serve a person throughout life. Words are used for communication, but they also facilitate a person's cognitive processes. Words can be produced in a spoken form, but also in written form, and, within AAC, as output of a speech-generating device. Instead of words, lexical equivalents are often used in AAC. These include graphic symbols and manual signs (see Chapter 4). Very often, in AAC, decisions need

to be made as to the size of the lexicon, how to structure the lexicon, and to which words one should give priority.

ZIPF'S LAW, CORE VOCABULARIES, AND AAC

Words are a source of fascination for psycholinguists, educators, and speech-language pathologists. On the one hand, it is clear that many people have the potential to know many words, but on the other hand, it is also clear that not all words are as frequent. This latter phenomenon is described in Zipf's law (after the linguist George Zipf, 1935): the frequency of a word is inversely related to its ranking on the frequency list. This means that the second word on the list has half the frequency of the first word, and that the first word is three times as frequent as the third word (Levelt, 2013). Simply put, the most frequent words are, well, really frequent. Therefore, it is not surprising that many practitioners in AAC have argued that the focus should be on establishing a core vocabulary (i.e., a relatively limited lexicon with a high degree of functionality). At the same time, AAC users should not be deprived from access to all the lexical elements that they are mentally able to manage. The issue is essentially about how to strike the right balance between quick access to a core lexicon and a more extended lexicon that will require more operations to access.

TYPICAL WORD DEVELOPMENT

Typical children learn new words at an incredibly fast pace. Developmental psychologists talk about the "vocabulary spurt," which occurs between the ages of 18 months and 5 years. According to some estimates, children will "know" 14,000 words by the time they are in kindergarten (Clark, 1993). Note that we use the term "knowing words" in a somewhat loose way as it is not always clear from the literature how "knowledge" is measured. Furthermore, one needs to be careful when talking about the number of words a person knows. Are "house" and "houses" the same word (in a different morphological environment), or are they two different words? What about "go" and "went," do

they count as one or two words? These and other questions have more relevance for AAC than might appear at first sight. We discuss this later in this chapter.

However, the development and growth of a person's vocabulary (their lexicon) does not stop at the age of 5 or 6. The lexicon keeps growing and developing, possibly during your entire life. Your grandmother may well have the following words in her lexicon: microwave, computer, iPod, compact car, texting, and many more that were not "available" when she was a young girl. Recently, I talked to a computer-savvy person who emigrated as a young adult from Russia to the United States (in the early 1990s). She told me that, although she remains fluent in Russian (her native language), she has trouble talking about topics related to computers and electronic communication. A whole new vocabulary has emerged and has been adopted by a whole generation of users of all ages (not just those who are in the middle of their language acquirement). New words are learned throughout one's entire life. However, the growth of the lexicon is most impressive in children. Estimates vary from source to source, but all estimates indicate that children must have an impressive capacity for quickly acquiring words.

QUESTIONS REGARDING VOCABULARY AND AAC

There are a number of questions that arise in regards to lexical development that are relevant to AAC: (1) Through which mechanism(s) do typical children learn new words?, (2) How do typical children organize their lexicon to facilitate access?, and (3) What is the relation between lexical and syntactic development? We come back to these questions below.

Typical adult language users have enormous lexicons. Estimates are that adults can have mental access to more than 100,000 words (Lorge & Chall, 1963). Obviously, there are varying ways to measure and estimate this number. For example, a distinction can be made between a receptive lexicon and a productive lexicon (a distinction that is not without importance in the context of AAC). Furthermore, estimates differ depending on whether one counts morphologically derived forms as distinct words (e.g., are "kind" and "kindly" two words, or two forms of the same word?). Everything indicates that humans have an amazing capacity to learn and use an incredible number of words. This growth occurs in a natural, spontaneous way One would expect that AAC intervention be focused on making words available so that the user can absorb and use them. Interestingly, AAC practitioners and researchers are often more concerned with issues such as: (1) selecting a vocabulary for AAC users and (2) teaching techniques for vocabulary.

Do practitioners worry about the wrong issues? Is there a reason to believe that AAC users have less lexical capacity than the general population? The answer is: yes and no. AAC users have a number of potential challenges when it comes to acquiring and using a lexicon. Here are a few:

1. Some AAC users are at a developmental level of beginning communicators —they need an initial lexicon. What should such a lexicon look like? And where should it start?
2. AAC users are often limited by the number of lexical elements and by the ways they can be accessed physically. How can we ensure easy access to a person's own lexicon?
3. Educators may unintentionally limit the person's acquisition by assuming a limited capacity. Who influences lexical growth? What words should one put on the devices? What expressions?
4. Lexical development of a person may have to be measured in a nonspeech modality.
5. The relation between words and manual signs is complicated. Because a manual sign uses metaphors and characteristics in the visual-gestural modality, it may contain connotations that are different from the spoken word.
6. The relation between words and graphic symbols is complicated. If "a picture is worth a thousand words," would that mean that "knowing one picture" would equal the knowledge of multiple words?
7. AAC users have to do more with less. Because lexical access often requires extra effort and time, AAC users will naturally seek to economize on word use.

Let's focus on each of these challenges and try to explore what they mean for lexical development and AAC.

1. Some AAC users are at the developmental level of beginning communicators—they need an initial lexicon. What should it look like?

In typical language development, the first lexicon of 50 words is acquired during the second year of life (Dale & Goodman, 2005). After this point, the so-called vocabulary spurt occurs (i.e., several years of acquiring new words, through different processes related to quick incidental learning). The first 50-word lexicon has received much attention from researchers, as it is believed that it constitutes a set of functionally distinct elements, serving and ensuring the child's most basic needs. It seems that the first set of 50 words serves as a launching base for development. It is something that requires more care, time, and effort to build up, and afterward children go on to learn fast.

Indeed, when describing the initial lexicon of normal developing children, we encounter words (or some equivalents) such as mommy, daddy, night-night, more, bye-bye, hi, doggy, bath, as well as sound imitating idiosyncratic words such as mm-mm (I am hungry), or vroom vroom (for car). It is important to realize that these first words constitute a set that enables the child to pragmatically function in a baby world. Initially, it has a strong emphasis on behavior regulation words, words related to basic functions, and words referring to the child's primary caregivers. As a child progresses in word acquisition, the need for these basic-type words may decrease. Snow (1988) states that there is a functional difference between the first and the tenth word, as there is a difference between the tenth and the twentieth word. Pragmatic needs and needs for new words to be learned evolve as the child learns and acquires more.

Much attention has been given to initial functioning for prelinguistic communicators and communicators at the transition from prelinguistic to linguistic communicative use (see Chapter 6). It makes sense that many educators and clinicians propose to start with "a request lexicon," allowing users to indicate that they want to have their preferred food or that they need to go to the bathroom, or another basic function. In general, it

is good practice to let the initial lexicon "grow" with the needs and preferences as they are observed throughout a person's daily life. However, one needs to be aware of two risks: (1) the risk that we might not "see" specific needs, or (2) the risk that we don't go "beyond requesting" (i.e., that users only learn to ask for things or activities, but that they are insufficiently taught or encouraged to use other communicative functions such as rejection, socializing, or commenting).

As for the need to see "all" the needs of the person, it is important to realize that the ability to request should always go together with the ability to reject or refuse. If clinicians and educators solely focus on requesting, it can happen that the users have to resort to problem behavior (i.e., screaming, temper tantrums, aggression, running away, etc.) when they are not happy about what is happening or what is presented to them. Therefore, it is important to include words (signs, symbols) to indicate "no," "stop," "I don't like it," and so on. If we look at communication from a functional angle, this all makes sense; communication is a means to facilitate a good quality of life. Therefore, they need to be able to request what they need as well, as they need to be able to tell that there is something that they don't want. Rejection is as important as requesting. Refusal and rejection are also important for another reason. We should realize that individuals with severe communicative limitations are among the most likely to be victimized through a whole range of abuses (including verbal abuse, neglect, physical abuse, financial abuse, and sexual abuse). Unfortunately, being limited in communication makes it harder to report abuse or even to signal that one does not agree with another person's decisions or behavior. Abuse can and does happen with the most vulnerable of all: those who have the most limited communication repertoire. Therefore, communication intervention needs to make it possible to "say no." Not only does rejecton need to be represented on the communication device (or in the lexicon taught) but it also needs to be part of awareness-raising education about trust and careful behavior toward strangers, specific requests, and specific behaviors.

How do you go beyond requesting? It is essential to make sure that the lexicon contains a growing number of: (1) social interaction words and (2) possibilities to comment. Social interaction lexical items can include words as "fun," "hello," "thank you," "please," and "nice." Possibilities to comment include labeling of persons, animals, toys, things, and events that matter and that play a role in the life of the person. It includes real elements such as a teddy bear, the sibling's name, the television set, but also qualifiers such as "good," "yellow," "big," and fictitious characters from picture books.

The first lexicon will be small and grow slowly. Provide the learners with sufficient numbers of new words. Remember, normally developing speaking children surprise us all the time with new words that they have picked up here and there. Who can predict what the first 50 words of a child will be? One of the first 50 words of a normal child might be "calendar" because that is what she could have heard when people where pointing to the colorful picture on the wall. AAC users often do not have the choice to learn words other than those that have been "planned" to be taught, or those that have been programmed into the communication device. Therefore, it seems better to expose users to more words than they can learn and absorb. This appears to be

preferable to posing limitations on the number of words they can learn.

2. AAC users are often limited by the number of lexical elements and by the ways they can be accessed physically. How can we ensure easy access to a person's own lexicon?

How many symbols can go on a communication board or a screen? Although an internal mental lexicon may have an unlimited capacity, it is hard to place an unlimited number of lexical elements onto one communication board or display. Although we should be happy that our clients know and want to use many lexical elements, it is clear that representing many of them on one screen or on one board would be impossible to manage.

This is a problem of lexical organization. Educators and clinicians have tried to solve this problem with nontech solutions such as the use of several communication boards (for different situations: classroom, home, schoolbus), or the use of a binder. The problem is addressed in high technology in a number of ways: (1) through dynamic screens, (2) through icon sequencing, and (3) through visual scene displays.

Let's review how nondisabled speakers use their mental lexicon. Speakers can easily speak two to three words a second (Levelt, 1989). This means that they are able to access their lexicon, identify the word that is needed, and activate the word into articulated speech in an amazingly fast way. Speed of mental access is of the essence to ensure successful spoken communication. This is only possible because speakers have well-organized internal lexicons, and because navigating through the mental lexicon is usually fast and efficient. Psycholinguistic research shows that the "mental search engine" (when we are trying to find words) uses multiple cues to find words. In the first place, words are stored according to semantic principles (Murray & Forster, 2004). Psycholinguists study this through priming. In word priming, participants are asked to read words that are flashed on a computer screen and to push a button as soon as they recognize the word. Shortly after a first word is flashed (for example "house"), another word appears. If the new word is semantically related to the first word (for example "street") individuals respond faster (measured in milliseconds) than if the word is unrelated (say "guitar"). This indicates that lexicons are organized according to semantic principles. Interestingly, words that are not related semantically but that are similar in other ways (e.g., they have the same number of syllables or they have the same word beginning) also yield faster reaction times. It appears thus that the mental lexicon is a very flexible internal database that is easily accessible according to semantic, syntactic, and phonological principles.

If we want AAC to work, we will need to organize the lexicon in a way that allows fast access. How well are we doing this now? Much is left to be desired, that is certain. The nontech approaches are certainly failing us. Organizing words and symbols in binders and on communication boards is sometimes the best option, but it is certainly not an option that allows for fast access. Most of the time, words and symbols are placed on pages according to themes (e.g., bedtime) or to locations (classroom) and requires good understanding of the communicative situation to know which words go where. Often educators (and the users) find themselves confronted with the dilemma of choosing between a few fast-accessible words or many symbols that require (too much) time to access.

High-tech devices can do a better job in simulating a real mental lexicon. In the first place, they can let the user "navigate" through screens (often called dynamic displays). Screens can be personalized and built up as the vocabulary grows. Words (or messages) are stored in specific places. Users navigate through the screens to "find" the word. When you compare this with the natural "word finding" process, you can see right away why this is still challenging. First, you have to remember where the words are stored. Compare this with how nondisabled people speak and access their words, without having any idea that the words that one produces are actually stored somewhere. Second, you need to steer the device toward the word (this can be done with any type of physical access mode: touching, clicking a mouse, eye gazing, etc.). The speed with which the device responds will depend on factors related to the software and the hardware. It is clear that finding and managing words in a communication device (low-tech or high-tech) requires more time and more metalinguistic effort than normal speech.

Of course, there is an alternative to storing word by word in the device and requiring the person to find the entire word in a location. That alternative is the combinatorial principle. This principle states that individuals tend to prefer to assemble their messages and their words "on the fly." The best example is probably writing or typing. When you type, you are not looking up entire words but you assemble the parts of the words (the letters) as you are producing your message. Typing is certainly not as fast as natural speech, but it relieves the user from putting too much cognitive effort in locating the words. Learning to type is a form of motor learning, where the user masters psychomotor patterns that "take over" the cognitive effort (ask an experienced typist where on the keyboard the letter "p" is. Chances are that they have to "type in the air" to give you the answer.). Experienced literate AAC users know this. They often prefer to use a letter-board or a communication device that has a typewriter-type input, linked to speech output (Figure 5–1).

This observation is a strong argument in favor of placing emphasis on literacy learning for children and individuals who are AAC users. It is only in the past 15 years that literacy has been recognized as a crucial clinical and educational objective for AAC users (this is discussed in more detail in a later chapter).

However, full literacy is not always achieved or achievable for every AAC user. Nevertheless, this doesn't mean that the combinatorial principle cannot be used. Bruce Baker, one of the earliest pioneers within AAC, designed Minspeak that allows the user to com-

bine icons to produce words. This principle is called icon sequencing. With one screen of 84 or 128 icons, the user can, in principle, generate an infinite number of messages (see Chapter 2).

The user will no longer have to remember the location of the symbols and the words; no time wasted with navigating, but instead will have to remember the combinatorial code. Although there is ample evidence that both young and older learners can master the system (often without being literate), there are not many studies that explore the processes involved in the use of an icon sequencing system compared with a navigation system.

3. Educators may unintentionally limit the person's acquisition by assuming a limited capacity. Who influences lexical growth? What words should one put on the devices? What expressions?

Most of the words that typical speakers know and use are not the result of a teaching process. Speakers pick up most of the words in natural and interactive contexts. Most parents never think of which words need to be taught and learned. And maybe that is a good thing. Most parents would never have the time to teach their children thousands of words. It would probably never occur to parents that they would have to explicitly teach their children words such as "grin," "prompt," "sob," and most of what you find in the dictionary. In general, children (and adults) acquire the words when these present themselves in a meaningful context. It is probably not bad that we don't have to leave it to parents to offer their children a "vocabulary curriculum." However,

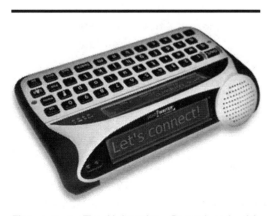

Figure 5–1. The Lightwriter. Reproduced with permission from Dynavox.

that is what we often have to do in AAC. Educators, parents, and clinicians need to program the devices, and write or insert words and symbols on communication boards and binders.

There are many discussions about which words to be used in devices. Often a distinction is made between core vocabulary and fringe vocabulary. *Core vocabulary* consists of words that can be used in multiple contexts by many language users. These are the lexical indispensables. *Fringe vocabulary* consists of words that are specific for an individual, containing words that refer to objects, persons, or events that are relevant to specific contexts. The distinction is useful in determining which words to include in communication tools and devices depending on the situation (e.g., mealtimes; Balandin & Iacono, 1999), classroom lessons, or home situations. Other terms used include coverage vocabulary to indicate words that are needed to cover essential messages and developmental vocabulary, containing words that are not yet known but that will be added to the system to foster vocabulary growth.

Sometimes, clinicians and researchers refer to studies about the frequency of the use of words in children or in the general population. For example, Banajee and colleagues (Banajee, Dicarlo, & Stricklin, 2003) noted that the following words were among the most frequent used by toddlers: I, no, yes, want, it, that, my, you, more. Similarly, according to Wiktionary, the 100 most frequent words in TV and movie scripts are: "a · about · all · and · are · as · at · back · be · because · been · but · can · can't · come · could · did · didn't · do · don't · for · from · get · go · going · good · got · had · have · he · her · here · he's · hey · him · his · how · I · if · I'll · I'm · in · is · it · it's · just · know · like · look · me · mean · my · no · not · now · of · oh · OK · okay · on · one · or · out · really · right · say · see · she · so · some · something · tell · that · that's · the · then · there · they · think · this · time · to · up · want · was · we · well · were · what · when · who · why · will · with · would · yeah · yes · you · your · you're." There are almost no nouns in the list —most of the words are conjunctions that function as the cement between the real content words. In AAC, clinicians generally agree that one needs to make nouns as the most prominent words on devices. Maybe this unveils that the use of frequency lists taken from nondisabled communicating individuals might be a flawed approach. As discussed throughout this chapter, nondisabled people have ready and fast access to thousands of words—which make speech production a rapid process. This allows spoken language to have a high degree of redundancy, often expressed in the small words (I, you, that). In situations where speakers have to weigh effort and rapidity of what to say, they are more likely to switch to different strategies—choosing high-meaning words (nouns!) as these provide us generally with a better effort—effect ratio.

4. Lexical development of a person may have to be measured in a nonspeech modality.

How do we really know how many words a person knows? In general, we use estimates. Most speakers understand more words than they actually use in a productive way. There is a discrepancy between the number of words we "know" passively (we understand them), and the number of words that are part of our active vocabulary. The active vocabulary consists of the words that you internally can access and subsequently activate into speech. Vocabulary tests take that into account. When we think of individuals who use AAC, it is obvious that the situation is quite different. First of all, AAC users may be able to mentally access words in their internal lexicon, but may be hindered in their expression because: (1) the word is not available on the board or the device and (2) if available, it takes too much time and effort to physically access it (navigate the system) and activate it.

Observers (including clinicians) may get the wrong impression of a low lexical potential of a child because there is so little diverse speech output. One needs to keep in mind that the active word output by AAC users is probably a far shadow from what their real word knowledge is and what their potential is. One of the gravest errors that we can make is to "feed less words into the person's system" (i.e., expose them to fewer words) because we think they can only handle a limited number.

To get an idea of the person's lexicon, the passive vocabulary may be the more reliable indicator. The best thing to do is to observe if the person understands words and is able to respond adequately to words.

---

5. The relation between words and manual signs is complicated. Because a manual sign uses metaphors and characteristics in the visual–gestural modality, it may contain connotations that are different from the spoken word.

The sign languages of deaf communities are real and full-fledged languages. This means that they have all the critical linguistic components, including phonology (a combinatorial system of sublexical elements—the phonemes), morphology (small meaningful elements), syntax, and a lexicon. The phonemes of sign languages are the basic formational aspects (i.e., the sign movement, the place at or close to the body where the sign is made, and the hand configuration that makes the sign). However, despite the structural similarities, signed and spoken languages do have differences. A spoken language uses acoustic signals, and a sign language uses visual signals. Humans process acoustic signals through the ear and visual signals through the eye. Visual and auditory perceptions are not the same. This is reflected in the way both types of languages have structured their phonology, morphology, and syntax. Spoken languages are mainly structured in a sequential way (the phonemes are in a sequence) while sign language contains a stronger simultaneous component (e.g., the hand configuration, the movement, and the place of articulation of the sign are activated at the same time).

Manual Sign Lexicons

Fristoe and Lloyd (1980) were among the first to propose an initial sign lexicon, largely based on principles of functionality and ease of performance.

It is important to remember that AAC users only seldom use sign language. Most of the time they may use manual signing (i.e., they use manual signs that have been borrowed, with or without adaptations, from the natural sign languages used in deaf communities). In AAC use, signs are employed either as stand-alone expressions (a single sign—e.g., MORE—to express that you want more of something, or that you want an activity or event to continue) or in combination with other communication modalities, often in a form of key word signing (Windsor & Fristoe, 1991). The syntactic structures and sign order of a sign language is seldom practiced in AAC.

However, the individual signs still can carry some of the specific characteristics of a sign language. Signs can have simultaneous modulations to express notions for which most spoken languages would use several words. For example, one would sign "big ball" by simply modifying the size of the sign, rather than using two signs, big and ball. Klima and Bellugi (1979) were among the first to describe the rich inflectional system of American Sign Language that through small (but systematic) modulations of the same sign can distinguish "sick" from "get sick" and "prone to sickness," as well as the fact that "chair" and "to sit" are two different modulations of the same sign. Sign languages invest more in simultaneous modulations, which makes it possible to save on the number of words. Depending on how you count, the size of the lexicon of sign languages may vary. Do you count "to look" and "to stare" as one or as two different signs? (Both have the same basic form, but "to stare" is performed with a slightly longer static position.) It may not matter that much, as long as we understand where the differences come from. Likewise, an AAC person who uses manual signs may know and use more signs that we tend to count. Once the person understands the principle of modulation, they may be able to discover that you can do "come here" and "go there" with the same underlying sign. The same is true for modulations such as happy and very happy, surprised, startled, and many more.

6. The relation between words and graphic symbols is complicated. If "a picture is worth a thousand words" would knowledge and use of a few graphic symbols match the knowledge of more words?

In Chapter 4, we discussed *polysemy*, the phenomenon that words have multiple meanings. We mentioned that this could be confusing when we try to decide which graphic symbols to use. When we think of the size of a person's lexicon, one may wonder if *fan* (as in "*he is a big fan of that rock star*") and *fan* (as in "*thanks to the fan on the ceiling, we got some fresh air*") is one single word or two. If you use graphic symbols, things become more complicated. Take for example the graphic symbol in Figure 5–2.

You may be able to use this symbol for one meaning of the English word *fan*, but you would probably resist using this to indicate that you are a fan of the Dave

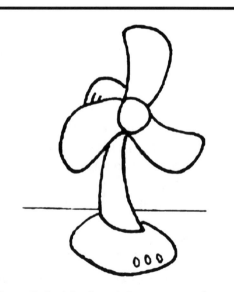

Figure 5–2. A fan is not always a soccer fan.

Matthews band. The picture qualities of the graphic symbols sets limits on the semantic scope. For example, when you see a picture of a wind-producing device, it is much less likely to activate the meaning of the music fan(-atic).

Does this indicate that words have more meanings than graphic symbols? Not at all! There are many graphic symbols that can be used for multiple meanings (just like the same manual sign can have multiple meanings). What meanings can we give to the picture in Figure 5–3? It can mean roof, chimney, house, home, gutter, and one might be able to come up with even more derived or associated meanings, such as coziness, protection, or shelter.

What is the point of all this? The point is that there is not an identical relationship between words and meanings as there is between graphic symbols and meanings. In fact, this is not only the case

for graphic symbols and English words. Many linguists emphasize that it is almost impossible to find an exact counterpart of most of the words in two languages. Take the word "ball" in English. If you look it up in an English-French dictionary, you find that the translation is "ballon." But "ballon" is also a translation of "balloon." At the same time, if we want to go for a dance you can go to "a ball" in English, but you shouldn't go to a "ballon" in French. No dancing in a "ballon."

What is the moral of all this? That we need to be careful in interpreting the significance of a person's knowledge of words, manual signs, and graphic symbols. Maybe, instead of just focusing on counting the number of words that a person knows, we might do better to focus on the number of concepts and ideas a person is having, and . . . if we are able to give the person the means to express these ideas—through AAC.

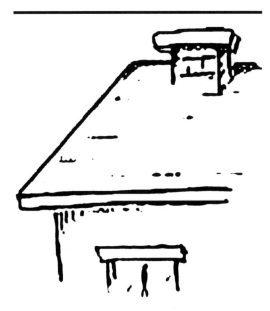

Figure 5–3. Home, roof, protection, and more: The same picture can refer to many words.

7. AAC users have to do more with less. Because lexical access often requires extra effort and time, AAC users will naturally seek to economize on word use.

The problems of AAC users in using their lexicon include: (1) the physical access to the lexical elements, and (2) the speed of processing (navigating through the device may just be asking too much).

Interestingly enough, when we see AAC users communicating, they come up with strategies to do the best possible. Once I saw an AAC user who asked me about the "Bruce Conference" to indicate the Pittsburgh Employment Conference, organized by Bruce Baker. Intervention should be encouraging these creative linguistic solutions that arise out of necessity (because the user needs to come up with a solution if the words are not available or if they would require too much navigation). Intervention should also help the AAC user to find shortcuts within the device.

Finally, "How to select a lexicon for an AAC user" is a question that is heard often in debates and publications. Maybe it is the wrong question. It suggests that the lexicon is chosen and directed by a caregiver, and educator, a clinician, or a parent. However, that is not what parents of typically developing children do. If parents had to select a lexicon for their children (instead of giving them ample and continuous opportunities to discover and learn new words incessantly), all children (hence also adults) would end up with a meager lexicon. Let's not make this error with children who are AAC users. Let's give them new words, put them in the device or on the communication board—but give them all the chances in the world to learn the thousands of words that help them in their thinking.

CONCLUSION

In typical development, most of language is acquired. It is learned, not taught. Typically developing children have an impressive capacity to acquire a language. Children with developmental limitations may not be able to acquire language as fast and thoroughly as typical children. AAC can be an aid to let them explore the world. It can offer a modality that increases access for the user. However, because caregivers often play a role in "providing" the lexicon, there are risks that the lexicon may not be commensurate with the person's natural lexical growth, preferences, and needs. This needs to be taken into consideration in intervention planning.

POINTS TO REMEMBER

- In AAC, the issue is about how to strike the right balance between quick access to a core lexicon and a more extended lexicon that will require more operation to access.
- As in typical language development, an initial lexicon for AAC users needs to contain words that serve a multitude of functions in the daily life of the user.
- Educators need to be aware of the fact that AAC users may experience constraints by the selection of lexical elements available in the AAC system.
- Graphic symbols and words do not have a one-on-one semantic relation. The same is true for the relation between manual signs and words.
- Lexical development of a person may have to be measured in a nonspeech modality.
- AAC users have to do more with less. Because lexical access often requires extra effort and time, AAC users will naturally seek to economize on word use.

REFERENCES

Balandin, S., & Iacono, T. (1999). Crews, wusses, and whoppas: Core and fringe vocabularies of Australian meal-break conversations in the workplace. *AAC: Augmentative and Alternative Communication, 15*(2), 95–109 (66 ref).

Banajee, M., Dicarlo, C., & Stricklin, S. B. (2003). Core vocabulary determination for toddlers.

AAC: Augmentative and Alternative Communication, 19(2), 67–73 (23 ref).

Clark, E. V. (1993). *The lexicon in acquisition.* Cambridge, UK: Cambridge University Press.

Dale, P. S., & Goodman, J. C. (2005). Commonality and individual differences in vocabulary growth. In M. Tomasello & D. I. Slobin (Eds.), *Beyond nature and nurture: Essays in honor of Elizabeth Bates* (pp. 41–78). Mahwah, NJ: Lawrence Erlbaum Associates.

Dunn, M., & Dunn, L. M. (2007). *The Peabody Picture Vocabulary Test—4.* Circle Pines, MN: AGS.

Fristoe, M., & Lloyd, L. L. (1980). Planning an initial expressive sign lexicon for persons with severe communication impairment. *Journal of Speech and Hearing Disorders, 45*(2), 170–180.

Klima, E. S., & Bellugi, U. (1979). *The signs of language.* Cambridge, MA: Harvard University Press.

Levelt, W. J. M. (1989). *Speaking: From intention to articulation.* Cambridge, MA: The MIT Press.

Levelt, W. J. M. (2013). *A history of psycholinguistics: The pre-Chomskyan era* (1st ed.). Oxford: Oxford University Press.

Lorge, I., & Chall, J. (1963). Estimating the size of vocabularies of children and adults: An analysis of methodological issues. *The Journal of Experimental Education, 32*(2), 147–157.

Murray, W. S., & Forster, K. I. (2004). Serial mechanisms in lexical access: The rank hypothesis. *Psychological Review, 111*(3), 721–756.

Snow, C. (1988). The last word: Questions about the emerging lexicon. In M. Smith & J. Locke (Eds.), *The emergent lexicon* (pp. 341–352). San Diego, CA: Academic Press.

Windsor, J., & Fristoe, M. (1991). Key word signing: Perceived and acoustic differences between signed and spoken narratives. *Journal of Speech and Hearing Research, 34*(2), 260–268.

Zipf, G. K. (1935). *The psycho-biology of language. An introduction to dynamic philology.* Boston, MA: Houghton-Mifflin.

CHAPTER 6

AAC Intervention at the Prelinguistic Level

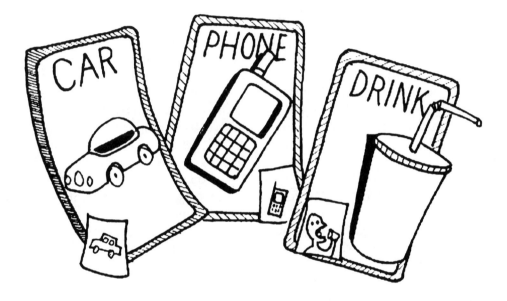

Since the early days that AAC became a recognized and established applied discipline, it was never called into question that it could serve individuals who had *acquired* language and linguistic skills. However, the realization that AAC could be useful for individuals functioning at a prelinguistic level took a while to be accepted. In the past, practitioners and educators have sometimes shown hesitance or reluctance to introduce AAC at an early developmental level, based on the assumptions: (1) that developmental prerequisites needed to be met before AAC intervention would work or (2) that the introduction of alternative modalities would prevent the development of natural forms of communication. As Kangas and Lloyd already pointed out in 1988, these views are inaccurate and developmentally counterproductive (Kangas & Lloyd, 1988; see also Romski & Sevcik, 2005). Today's perspectives are different: Even typically developing children start with nonspeech communication (e.g., eye gaze, interactions, gesture), which paves the way toward linguistic communication. These insights have lent legitimacy and evidence for the use of AAC with infants and toddlers with disabilities (Branson & Demchak, 2009).

In typical language acquisition, the first words appear around the child's first birthday (Gaskell & Ellis, 2009). Around 18 months, children start to combine words, which can be seen as the first forms of syntactic structures (Tomasello, 2009). Thus, it takes about one year in typical children for linguistic communication to kick in. This does not mean that children are not paying attention or learning language in the first 12 to 18 months. On the contrary, the prelinguistic period is entirely a communicative period. What the child learns in these crucial months is the basis for communication and language development.

AAC starts here. AAC may provide solutions that help the first steps toward communication and toward language for young children with severe developmental limitations. A developmental perspective provides a framework for a rationale for both early AAC intervention (Cress & Marvin, 2003) and intervention at all ages for individuals functioning at a prelinguistic level, for whom AAC can contribute to quality of life.

In this chapter, we: (1) first describe a developmental framework to understand the early development of interaction toward communication and language, then (2) use this framework to suggest AAC solutions for early intervention and school intervention. Finally, (3) we discuss how these solutions can be applied to people with severe developmental limitations of all ages.

THE BEGINNINGS OF COMMUNICATION

When does communication start? Despite what people may think, communication appears long before children utter their first words. Through crying, smiling, and other behaviors, children communicate with their caretakers from early on. Through this communicative behavior parents and caretakers come to "understand" or at least interpret what their children are trying to say (Bornstein & Tamis-LeMonda, 2010). Do parents and caregivers really understand what babies are trying to say? Do babies really attempt to tell/communicate with us? Do they have the intention to say something? Could we just be reading too much into their behaviors?

These questions reflect a major part of what research into early communication of typical (and atypical) children is trying to discover. Obviously, it all depends on how you interpret the term "communication." What is communication? Harley (2008, p. 54) describes communication as "the transmission of a signal that conveys information." If we accept this definition, then communication starts on day one in a person's life. Newborn babies can "communicate" that they are awake, that they are asleep, that they are male or female, and more.

Likewise, all individuals communicate all kinds of information (mainly about themselves) without much being aware of it: our gender, our physical appearances, maybe the mood that we are in, our clothing preferences, and our age (there is only so much you can do when it comes to lying about your age). Much of this information is, of course, unintentional. People "give away" clues about their state of mind, their background, their cultural habits and behaviors.

"One cannot not communicate" is an axiom made famous by the psychologist and philosopher Paul Watzlawick (Watzlawick, Bavelas, & Jackson, 1967). If we apply this to newborn babies, children in the prelinguistic stage, and individuals with severe communication limitations, we have a promising basis to start from: every person does display communicative behavior, on which we could build more advanced and more effective forms.

FORMS OF COMMUNICATION

What does a baby do to communicate? As it is initially unintentional communication, it will depend on how the environment responds. In other words, the question should be which behaviors: (1) elicit a response from the communication partners and (2) are therefore likely to be repeated. When we think of it, we end up with a very long list of possible behaviors including crying, smiling, staring, vocalizing, facial expressions. In short: any (any!) behavior has communicative potential. This remains so during a person's entire life. Admitted, specific forms of behavior (speaking, writing) serve primarily as communication forms, but all behaviors keep their communicative potential. From infancy to adulthood, all of the same behaviors (nonlinguistic, nonintentional) can be communicative; behaviors such as the way one talks, looks, and exhibits facial expressions (often unintentional), "give away" information about us throughout our life span.

Siegel and Wetherby (2006, p. 419) provide a list of behaviors that a baby can (and does) display during the first year of life. These include (but are not limited to): vocalizations, facial expressions, touching or manipulating objects, assuming positions, withdrawal, and aggressive or self-injurious behavior. However, the list of communicative forms is always incomplete. One should add: "any behavior."

Any behavior is potentially a communicative act. Maybe scratching my head will always indicate that I am very worried about something. In fact, these behaviors are largely idiosyncratic (i.e., they belong to a personalized nonconventionalized system).

FUNCTIONS OF COMMUNICATION

Most of the research discusses which behaviors of children and adults are communicative. Intervention also tries to figure out what to do to make communication better. But shouldn't we also pay attention to *why* we communicate as well? What is the purpose of communication? When I ask this question to my students (or anybody) I almost always get an answer like, "to convey information," "to pass on my thoughts."

While this is certainly an important function, it is not the "first" function. To understand the purpose of communication, it helps to think in an evolutionary way (Tomasello, 2008). What makes us more likely to survive (especially when we are helpless babies)? Our survival and our safety is guaranteed: if (1) we can solicit the help from our environment for our most basic functions: food, safety, warmth, love, if (2) we feel accepted and taken care of by our environment, and if (3) our environment is willing to exchange information (that, in the long run, will make us more independent and able to protect ourselves).

In other words, these are the functions of communication: behavioral regulation, social interaction, and joint attention. Table 6–1 shows these behavioral categories as well as the evolutionary survival purpose.

Table 6–1. Communication Functions

Functions	What (Behavioral Categories)	Why (Survival Purpose)
Behavior regulation	Request Protest	Make sure that you are safe and that people take care of you
Social interaction	Request social routine Request comfort Greet Call Showing off Request permission	Make sure that you get attention, that you are protected, and loved by the environment. You show that you want to go by the social rules.
Joint attention	Comment about an object/ a person Request information	Build a system for information exchange

Behavior Regulation

When does a baby cry? When she is hungry, when she needs attention? Often the baby cries when she needs her caregivers to do something (feed her, change her diaper, etc.). Behavior regulation includes behavior categories such as requesting and rejecting. Not surprisingly, these are the topics that clinicians and educators will place on the first communication boards (I am hungry; I need to use the toilet, etc.). These requests are relevant to all individuals. For example, when adults travel to a foreign country, their first and main concerns are: "How do I ask for the bathroom?" "Where will I eat?" "Will they accept my money?" All of these questions are related to one's survival.

Social Interaction

However, it is important to assure the continued help and commitment of the people that take care of you. Therefore, establishing a personal contact (social interaction) through routines (e.g., in the feeding situation, during the changing of diapers) is vital! (Fiske, 2010). The drive to be part of, accepted by, and contributing to others in a person's environment is deeply engrained and drives the development of communication and its skills.

Joint Attention

Finally, you want to use this interpersonal connection to learn about the world (joint attention, information sharing)—as, in the long run, it will ensure you more independence and more chances of survival. Joint attention is the term used for situations and activities where communication results from a shared interest. In interactions with the youngest children, the interest is often initiated by the child (picking up a toy, looking at it, and vocalizing) who is then joined by the caregiver ("you like that rattle, don't you? Yes, you do!"—with all the typical intonation). This creates a triangular framework (Figure 6–1).

This joint attention framework is considered to be the prototype of any conversation that a person will have with another person during their life. Every conversation has this basic "me-you-something" structure, whether you comment on the weather, order a hamburger in a fast food restaurant, or discuss the future of technology with a group of experts. Establishing joint attention with young AAC users must be the central goal of intervention (Benigno, Bennett, Mccarthy, & Smith, 2012).

FROM UNINTENTIONAL BEHAVIOR TO INTENTIONAL COMMUNICATION

Let's go back to the typically developing young child. The first communication is unintentional communication—it is, in a sense, a one-way communication. Of course, as long as communication is unintentional, it may have limited value for intervention. Let's, therefore, take a look at the development of a typical child *from unintentional to intentional behavior*. It is believed that this largely is the result of: (1) understanding cause-effect, (2) the use of tools (instrumental use), and (3) the development of mental internal representations.

Understanding Cause–Effect

Cause-effect understanding arises gradually when children start to experience that "each time I do A, I notice that B happens." This is, in the theoretical framework of Piaget's developmental psychology, a sensory-motor understanding. It could be represented as the rule $A \rightarrow B$. This applies to the physical world around the child, and it includes the humans that the child interacts with. The rule $A \rightarrow B$ also applies to interactive behavior. For example, the child may figure out that "if I cry, they come and do something with me" (again, this is a sensory-motor awareness, not a verbal or even a conscious awareness), or "if I smile, they smile back, they pick me up, and start to talk funny to me. I like that." One can easily see how this gives rise to repetition and reinforcement. Parents reinforce the child to smile,

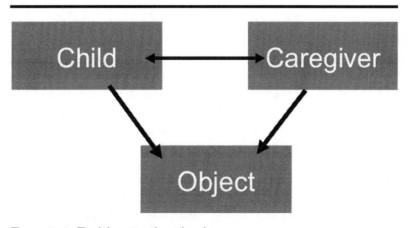

Figure 6–1. The joint attention triangle.

but the child also reinforces the parents to do so. We are somewhat in a reinforcement spiral.

The Use of Tools

When children are 8 to 10 months old, they start to understand the basics of physics. They understand that there are different routes to crawl from point A to point B (the direct route, but also the route by taking a detour if there is an obstacle on your way). Children also understand that you can use one object to push another and that you can touch something with a toy. You also discover that things may sound differently such as dropping a bear compared with dropping a cup. In these cases, you are using tools to obtain an effect. Elizabeth Bates (1976), a pioneering psychologist who has devoted her work to understanding how children learn and use language as communication, emphasizes that one of the major breakthroughs occurs when the child comprehends that words (and language) are social tools. The development of tool awareness in young children is a major milestone toward language use.

The Genesis of Internal Mental Representations

Language is often characterized as a system of internalized symbols. Piaget (1974) talked about the emergence of the semiotic function—the ability to represent through symbols—and observed that the first words, the first dreams (considered to be internalized images), and the beginning of symbolic play all occur in the same period

at the end of what he considered the sensory-motor developmental stage.

SYMBOL DEVELOPMENT

What helps children on their way toward acquiring symbols? Psychologists agree that *routines* in the life of the baby play an enormous role. Parents follow the same sequence of actions when they change diapers, when they feed the baby, and when they put the baby to bed. Routines are sequences of actions, a chain of events that is repeated multiple times (Tomasello, 1988). When you analyze the routine, you find a succession of smaller events. For example, every morning, after the caregiver dresses the baby, she picks her up in her arms. Picking up the baby is part of the larger routine, but the act of picking up can also be analyzed into smaller segments. The caregiver will hold her hands left and right of the baby, in order to pick her up. As a physical response to this, if the baby cooperates, she will move her arms slightly upward. This allows the caregiver to pick her up. Moving the arms upward then flows into reaching toward the caregiver. Over time, the baby will be able to "isolate" the reaching part of this sequence: stretching her arms will be a signal to indicate, "Pick me up."

What happens here is fascinating. Being picked up starts as a sequence of interaction (literally: action between people), between the child and the caregiver. The baby's arm-stretching is initially a physical response to the fact that the caregiver places her hands under the arms of the baby. The movement, however, changes into a signal and becomes the basis of a symbol that is understood by caregiver and baby. This is one example of how the first symbols (signals that are interpreted in the same way by at least two people) are rooted in sensory-motor actions, preferably interactions!

Routines are thus important for the early development of symbols. Think of a routine as a succession of segments where A leads to B, B leads to C, C leads to D, and the chain continues. If the sequence is always played in the same order, then A becomes a predictor of B, and B a predictor of C. Routines help us to build symbolic awareness and are, therefore, very important in the application of AAC for early communicators.

WHEN DOES COMMUNICATION BECOME LANGUAGE?

When exactly ends the prelinguistic developmental period? In other words, when does communication assume the characteristics of language? The prelinguistic development goes through the following subphases:

1. Interaction and communication are present from day one
2. Communication and interaction fosters symbol development
3. Symbol development leads to linguistic development

Or, to put it simply, interaction precedes communication, communication precedes symbol development, and symbol development precedes language development. But when can we call a symbol linguistic? A symbol can be considered to have reached linguistic value if: (1) it is conventionalized (if it is understood by others) and (2) it is part of a larger structural multilevel combinatorial system.

From Idiosyncratic to Conventionalized Symbols

The first symbols are idiosyncratic. However, by understanding what symbols do, children (and their partners) are at a breakthrough moment in communication development. Gradually, children get access to more conventionalized symbols —that is, behaviors that have an agreed-upon meaning, although they initially do not yet belong to a linguistic system. This is still the level of nonlinguistic symbolic communication. For example, many of the gestures that we use and understand are nonlinguistic. They are stand-alone meaningful symbols, but they are not subject to combinational rules such as those we have/found in language. Pointing, sighing, giggling, sticking out your tongue, picture use, are (or can be) symbolic, but are not part of language. In fact, the first words that children use are probably also stand-alone symbols. Although they are taken from language, they do not function as linguistic elements in the heads of the children. That only happens when children have a critical mass of words (maybe 50 or more) and when they can start to combine them and string them together into more complex utterances. That is when the transition from nonlinguistic symbolic communication to linguistic communication takes place.

Symbols Become Part of a Larger Structural Multilevel Combinatorial System

The discipline of developmental psycholinguistics attaches importance to the first combination of words as an indication that a child is acquiring a semantic-syntactic system (see e.g., Brown, 1973). Two-word utterances have been used as a guide to understand how children construct an initial internal grammar (Clark, 2009). In the past decades, research has shown that the combinatorial use of words is preceded and facilitated by the use of two-gesture combinations or gesture-word combinations (Capirci, Iverson, Pizzuto, & Volterra, 1996). This is important as it gives weight to the recommendations to use nonspeech symbols in combination with speech (Figure 6–2) and depicts four stages in the development from prelinguistic, unintentional communication to linguistic, conventionalized communication.

Read the figure from top to bottom and from left to right. Initially, all behavior is unintentional. The arrow to the right indicates that you continue to display unintentional behavior your entire life (you "give away" a lot of information about yourself all the time: your gender, your culture, your age, maybe your emotional state of the moment—if you are agitated, and so on). This is true for all four of the stages. In other words, a normal adult will display unintentional behavior, intentional nonsymbolic behavior (e.g. "approaching" someone to indicate you want to make contact), symbolic nonlinguistic behavior (gestures, pictures), and —of course—linguistic behavior (words).

AAC SOLUTIONS FOR EARLY INTERVENTION

When we work with individuals who have severe developmental limitations

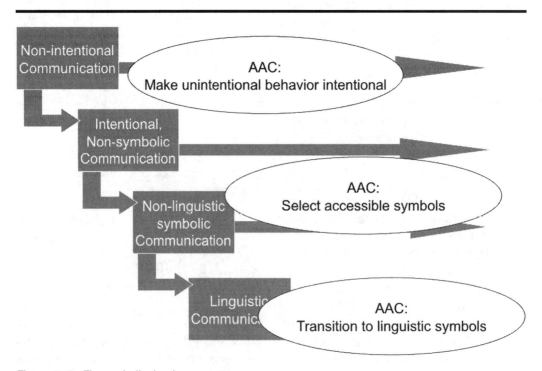

Figure 6–2. The symbolic development stages.

(i.e., who function at the prelinguistic level or at the level of beginning communicators), we need to: (1) assess the effectiveness of the existing communication system, (2) find the right AAC intervention to make prelinguistic communication as effective as possible, and (3) explore the possibilities to facilitate transition toward linguistic communication.

DETERMINING THE COMMUNICATION SYSTEM IN PLACE

Determining the communicative level and potential of individuals at the prelinguistic level is a tricky, sometimes complicated, and always idiosyncratic business. However, a careful analysis of the communication system in place can be a rich and strong basis for targeted intervention (see e.g., Braddock et al., 2012).

Keeping Watzlawick's axiom in mind ("One cannot not communicate"), we will need to determine and characterize the communication system that is already present. Talking to parents of children with severe developmental delays, I often heard comments like, "my child does not communicate at all." However, once you start talking to parents (or caregivers) and you ask question such as, "How does _____ (name of the person) let you know that he/she is hungry?," "Is there something in the behavior of _____ (name of the person) that tells you when he/she needs to use the bathroom?," and "Can you tell when _____ (name of the person) is upset," we always find that the parents (or caregivers) can answer these questions. Through such questions, parents and caregivers can be made aware of the fact that what

happens between them and the child is, in fact, what we call communication. Using a questionnaire that systematically explores the communication system (e.g., Snell & Loncke, 2005) that is already in place has enormous advantages. The use of a questionnaire helps shape an idea of the person's communication strengths and weaknesses. It also provides awareness for the child's parents or caregivers that they are indeed communicating with the child. Going through a questionnaire helps to realize that their child already has a communication system that has been developed in interaction with the caregivers. Although administering of such a questionnaire is essentially meant to gather information to start the intervention plan, it can be and should be regarded as a step in counseling the parents/caregivers on their role in communication intervention. Through talking with them and through the questions, parents and caregivers become aware that it is also *their* communication, and that what they do will have an impact on the quality of interaction. After all, communication is a shared phenomenon—we should not talk about "this client's communication," but about the "communication of this client and his/her partners."

The Learner

We should look at the prelinguistic communication from three angles: the person (the learner), the partner, and the environment. Under the *person*, we collect information that describes the skills and behaviors that are displayed by the client. Equally important (remember Bronfenbrenner's ecological model) are *the partners*. Here we focus on what partners do during the interaction, and how they approach and perceive the interaction. This brings us to the beliefs and the attitudes of the partners. The third component is *the environment*. How encouraging or how challenging is the environment? Remember that the first (and often the strongest) urges to communicate come from needs—hunger, thirst, and comfort. Are there challenges in the time schedule of the persons that make it necessary for them to communicate? Is everything predictable? (The more predictable things are, the less there is a need for communication.) Are there persons to communicate with (in some nursing homes, the work shifts of the caregivers are so hectic that there is no time for communication)?

Let's start with the assessment of the communication system that is in place. Through observations and through discussion with parents and caregivers, you can attempt to draft a description of this system. This could look like an inventory of *forms* and *functions*. You want to obtain a description and list of all the communication forms that a person uses. One way to do so is through the use of a questionnaire with parents or an observation scale (e.g., Fenson et al., 2007; Snell & Loncke, 2002; Wetherby & Prizant, 2002). Interviewing parents and daily interaction and communication partners is not wasted time—the information is extremely valuable (it usually shows you many places where you can start), and it helps in raising the partners' awareness of the issue.

If you want to make the prelinguistic communication richer and more effective, you will most likely have to start with the partners and the environment. For the *partners*, you will need to explore what they might want to try differently (e.g., changing the routines, using symbols, spending more time, talking to

the persons when they are attended to, etc.). For the *environment*, it may be helpful to discuss topics like: (1) identifying which persons are the preferred communication partners, (2) having favorite objects or toys, and (3) seeing if the routines can be altered to make them more communication-provoking.

The Partners

We already discussed how, in typical development, the child and the parents encourage each other in their communicative behavior. It is, therefore, extremely important to assess the partners' behaviors, perception, and beliefs toward communication with the child.

The Communicative Environment

You also need to assess the environment of the child (beyond the partners). Factors in the environment include the *time schedule* (e.g., how much time do nurses have to communicate with the client?), *opportunities and challenges* (e.g., does the person have a reason to communicate, or is everything preplanned and decided for them—clothing, food, and activities? Is the person given choices?

Once we have assessed the communication system that is in place, the role and habits of the communication partners, and the possibilities of the environment, we can focus on what we want to do in the intervention. For this we can go back to our figure describing the different levels of prelinguistic communication. This will give us indications of where AAC can help (Figure 6–3).

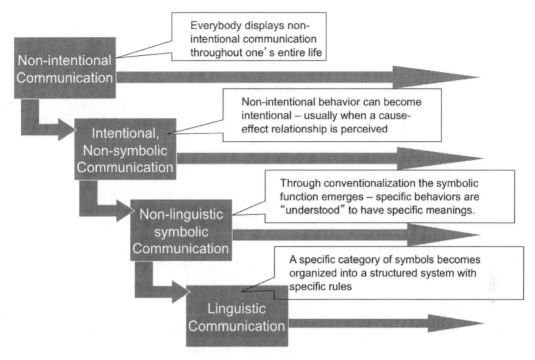

Figure 6–3. The symbolic development stages and AAC intervention.

Knowing that all behavior can assume communicative value is good news for AAC. In principle, AAC practitioners can identify behaviors "that work" for a specific person and take these as the starting point for the intervention. In AAC intervention, raising intentionality is an important goal. This is mainly done through routines where, often in a repetitive way, the child is given a reward when establishing a specific behavior. The team (the clinician together with the communication partners) needs to identify the behavior that will be communicative. Behaviors can be unaided (pointing, establishing

eye contact, vocalizing, a manual sign) or aided (activating a switch, hitting a one-message speech button). In determining which behavior you choose and want to reinforce, it is important to choose acceptable and nonproblem behaviors.

Identify Potential Communicative Acts

Sigafoos and collaborators (Sigafoos et al., 2000) proposed the term "potential communicative acts" to indicate behaviors that, through dynamic interaction, are candidates to become established signals between communicator and communication partners. These are behaviors to which partners respond in a consistent way (essentially by somehow indicating recognition) while the communicator grasps or imputes a meaning (i.e., a consequence) to the act. Based on observation, educators can select a behavior (e.g., eye contact) that they will consistently reward if produced in association with a specific context. For example, communication partners can systematically "shape" eye contact (looking the partner in the eye) into requesting behavior. (Braddock et al. [2013] have further explored this.)

Select Accessible Symbols

Symbols need to be physically and mentally accessible. *Physical accessibility* refers to the possibility by the person to physically produce the symbol by vocalization or by any voluntary action of their body (pointing, gesturing, grasping an object or symbol card, touching a screen, etc.). *Mental accessibility* is the cognitive effort to retrieve and understand the symbol. Gestures, graphic symbols, and some manual signs often appear to fall within the cognitive reach of individuals functioning at a prelinguistic level.

TRANSITION TO LINGUISTIC SYMBOLS

Although transition to linguistic functioning may not be a realistic goal for all individuals, prelinguistic intervention can facilitate entrance into basic language use for some. Research into the use of gestures in typical and atypical populations at least has shown that, although gestures (and other symbols) may not be internalized as linguistic symbols at their initial use,

they can grow into a linguistic-like mental network (Goldin-Meadow, 2009).

AAC APPLICATIONS FOR PEOPLE WITH SEVERE DEVELOPMENTAL LIMITATIONS OF ALL AGES

We tend to think of early communicators as babies and small children. However, individuals with severe developmental limitations may function at a prelinguistic level during their entire life. All the techniques discussed earlier may apply for clients of all ages. However, it is important to keep techniques chronologically age-appropriate—when determining routines, materials, and behaviors/symbols that will be used in intervention. Also, the partners will change over time. The school situation offers several opportunities (an environment focused on learning) and challenges (changing staff, teachers, less time to be devoted to one individual) than a family home situation. The same is true for adults, who might live in therapy homes or other settings (again, with their own opportunities and challenges).

For individuals of all ages, who function at the prelinguistic developmental level, AAC has two challenges: (1) make unintentional behavior intentional, and (2) make that behavior effective and acceptable. The two first functions on which we focus are *requesting* and *rejection*, the basic operations within behavior regulation! Teaching of requesting goes through enhancing awareness of intentionality. Again, it comes down to raising the awareness that "if I do this . . . they will do that." Olsson and Granlund (2003, p. 305) distinguish four levels of awareness of one's intention: unawareness of any intent, goal-intentional aware-ness, means-intentional awareness, and partner-intentional awareness.

> Level 1: Unawareness of any intent: the person displays behavior that does not reflect awareness of other people's behaviors.

> Level 2: Goal-intentional awareness: the person is focused on a goal, but there is no indication of understanding how to obtain the goal. For example, the person screams at seeing the food (that he can't reach) but has no strategy to get the food.

> Level 3: Means-intentional awareness: the person has learned that specific behaviors can be helpful. For example, a person with autism has learned that "making signs" sometimes will get you what you want. However, it is a random behavior—some kind of a trial and error.

> Level 4: Partner-intentional awareness: the person understands that the partner can play a role and that some kind of a relation needs to be established (by eye contact, taking the person's hand, etc.)

MAKE AND KEEP COMMUNICATION FUNCTIONAL

To determine priorities and goals for intervention (including AAC), it is now generally considered that a functional approach is essential. For example, the decision of insurance agencies for funding speech generating devices often depends on whether a convincing case can be made that the device will make a demonstrable difference for the person to communicate needs. It is also a recommendation made by educational departments (e.g., Virginia Department of Education Office of Spe-cial Education and Student Services, 2011) and it is a core concept within the Interna-tional Classification of Functioning, Dis-ability and Health (see Reed et al., 2005; see also Chapter 11).

ADDRESS PROBLEM BEHAVIOR

The terms "problem behavior" and "chal-lenging behavior" are used to refer to socially unacceptable or harmful behavior including aggression, self-injury, and tan-trums. Such behaviors may have devel-oped as a result of the fact that the indi-vidual experiences them as instrumental in obtaining attention from the environ-ment. For example, a child may have developed the habit of screaming when she is upset, when she wants something, even when she is happy. Over time, the screaming has obtained a generic com-municative meaning. Ironically, problem behaviors are often the most effective: they get you the attention of the environment. In other words, even the most motivated and well meaning parents and caregivers sometimes inadvertently encourage prob-lem behavior: they give the child atten-tion when he throws himself on the floor, when he screams, and certainly when he engages in self-injurious behavior. Clini-cians and educators need to work with the parents (and with each other) to discour-age (not reinforce) problem behavior and find communicative alternatives (Reichle & Wacker, 1993). A team can explore whether the child can learn to produce an acceptable behavior such as making a manual sign (or pointing to a picture) when he is upset (instead of the problem behavior). The replacement behavior will only be more effective if it gets as much attention—if the problem behavior is more effective, it will, sadly enough, persist. A functional analysis of the problem behavior (Repp & Horner, 1999; Walker & Snell, 2013) is useful to determine the purpose of the behavior and how to reduce or replace it by focusing on prevention and teaching new behaviors, including communication and coping skills. This includes a concrete description of the behavior, the situational contexts in which the behavior occurs, and conditions that maintain the challenging behavior (e.g., the consequences; Snell, Berlin, Voorhees, Stanton-Chapman, & Hadden, 2012).

forces the child to indicate that she wants to continue—what will she do? Will she come up with a signal? Will it be something that you can turn into a symbol?)

c. Offering a choice (you can "choose" through pointing, through gazing, and so on);

d. Presenting a familiar activity but with missing critical items (Will the child "protest" when she notices something is missing?);

e. Giving small portions of a favorite play material or food (The child may just look at you, but maybe will "do" something—it is the moment to introduce the behavior you want, maybe the manual sign for MORE);

f. Getting close to an individual who needs assistance but withholding assistance.

OTHER INTERVENTION TECHNIQUES

How do we encourage communication and early symbol development with low functioning individuals? Routines are certainly the way to go. Also, you could try to visualize your routines by making schedules and using graphic symbols. During the routines—as part of your intervention—one can use some of techniques that have been proposed by Wetherby and others (e.g., Wetherby & Prizant, 1989). These include:

a. Violating the expected sequence or outcome of a familiar routine and making a "silly situation" (for example, when dressing a child, you put the socks on the hands)

b. Pausing in the midst of an interesting spectacle or a favorite activity (this

REQUESTING AND REJECTING

With these "techniques," you try to modify the existing system (the routine) and challenge the child to do "something new."

Throughout this, we focus on teaching *requesting* and *rejection*. Sigafoos and Mirenda (2002), and others, discuss the use of AAC to gain and maintain access to preferred objects, activities, and actions, including requesting attention (Sigafoos, Drasgow, & Schlosser, 2003). It is essential that the intervention team define in a clear way which behavior is selected as the requesting behavior—and what the person can obtain with this behavior. It is crucial that all involved (the professionals as well as the daily communication partners) are aware of the importance of a systematic and sustained approach.

Teaching rejection may be a little trickier. Again, a behavior needs to be selected that will function and be recognized by all partners as having "rejection" as meaning (it can be shaking a head, but it can also be any other behavior). It is suggested to then modify the instructional environment of the person by creating the need to reject (offering choices that the person clearly does not want).

Beyond Requesting and Rejecting

In recent literature and research, there has been a concern that we risk that our interventions would not go "beyond requesting and rejecting." Therefore, one needs to plan social functions such as greeting, smiling, and communication through play. Gillette (2003) proposes to use a Communication Opportunities Inventory that measures an individual's independence in interacting, communicating, receiving information, and expressing information. This approach tracks communicative opportunities (and the behavior that is triggered, elicited, and prompted) in such natural situations as preparing and eating meals, shopping, watching television, making a bed, and getting dressed. This approach conforms to the general *functional* perspective on communication.

EXTENSION OF COMMUNICATIVE REPERTOIRE

Once a person has a small repertoire of meaningful behaviors (they may all still be nonsymbolic), one can consider if this repertoire can be extended. The best approach is through *dynamic assessment* (2002). Essentially, dynamic assessment

presents a person with small learning opportunities by introducing a new symbol, a new context, and a new challenge. By exploring (with the partners) what works and what could be learned by an individual, one can gradually introduce more symbols. Here again, it is imperative that all communication partners work together. One way of doing this is by keeping track of a "personalized" dictionary, a (growing) repertoire of what a person does, what it means, and how the partners should react (in order to encourage communicative development). Table 6–2 is an example of such a "dictionary" (from Snell & Loncke, 2002).

Educators and speech-language pathologists understandably wish to do everything possible to facilitate an individual's transition from the prelinguistic to the linguistic stage. Therefore, we are focused on teaching words, small spoken messages, and manual signs. All these come from languages—from linguistic systems. This is certainly a great goal and objective to remain focused on. However, true linguistic functioning may not always be a reachable goal (when dealing with people with severe developmental challenges). Working on more effective communication at a prelinguistic level can be a considerable contribution to the quality of life of clients. If one keeps a *dynamic assessment approach* (i.e., if one keeps exploring new ways that are learnable by the person), the individual's repertoire may grow naturally into a linguistic organization.

CONCLUSION

AAC techniques can and should be used to make pre-linguistic communication

Table 6–2. Communication Dictionary (from Snell & Loncke, 2002, 2005)

Jack's Communication Dictionary
Date: _____

What Jack does (signals)	What it means (functions)	What we do
Covers his ears	Too loud	Comment and turn noise down
Looks away	Not interested?	
Comes close, looks in your eyes	Interested	Comment, offer a choice, give a hug, explore what he wants
Makes "happy" noises while also looking at you	Interested wants something wants more?	Comment, offer a choice, give a hug, explore what he wants
Takes your hand and pulls it to something	Wants help	Comment and offer help
Hands you something	Wants help?	Comment and offer help
Looks at something, reaches for and maybe gets something, points and touches	Wants to hold/have the item	Comment and offer help
Makes sounds and looks unhappy	Dissatisfied with something	Try to figure out why he is unhappy
Hits himself; may also make unhappy noises	Wants activity to stop, wants to leave the situation, wants help; sometimes wants an object or activity?	Comment and offer help or stop/remove from activity; provide object/activity; ideally, we calm him, then prompt signal that means the same thing and fulfill request
Is aggressive to another person (scratches, pulls their hair)	Does not want the activity to continue; does not want the person to be there	Tell him no, possibly a very short time out, but when calm prompt better way to make request and fulfill it
Shakes head as if saying yes	May mean yes but also may be give me help or want more	Try to learn what he means
Picks up a picture or a symbol and hands it to you	He wants that item or more of that item	Comment and fill his request
Cries	Unhappy, does not feel good, tired, medication effect	Try to learn why he is unhappy

more effective. Based on the principle that there is always communication, a first step is to describe the communication system that is already in place. The communica-tion system is determined by the individ-ual learner, but also in major part by the communication partners (their responses and style), and by the environmental opportunities to communicate. Every behavior is potentially communicative. The environment can play a role in identifying behavior that can be shaped and reinforced into communicative behavior, and assume symbolic value. The intervention is geared at achieving effectiveness. It is possible that specific attention needs to be paid to avoiding or replacing unacceptable problem behavior.

POINTS TO REMEMBER

- There are no developmental prerequisites for the introduction of AAC at the prelinguistic level. AAC intervention can advance early communicative development.
- There is always communication. "One cannot not communicate" (Watzlawick). Therefore, it matters to assess and describe the earliest forms of communication.
- Early communication is idiosyncratic.
- Grasping cause–effect, the use of tools, and the development of internal representations, are three components that promote the development of symbolic skills.
- Early communicative intervention is geared at identifying "potential communicative acts," and solidifying emerging symbols.
- Any behavior can develop into a symbolic behavior.
- Conventionalization happens when communication partners accept and treat a behavior as carrier of a specific meaning.
- Early communication intervention is geared at achieving effectiveness, while avoiding, minimizing, or replacing problem behavior.

- A first step in pre-linguistic intervention is the description of the repertoire of communicative behaviors that is already in place.

REFERENCES

Assistive Technology Law Center. *AAC Report coach.* Retrieved from http://www.aacfundinghelp.com/report_coach.html

Bates, E. (1976). *Language and context: The acquisition of pragmatics.* New York, NY: Academic Press.

Benigno, J. P., Bennett, J. L., Mccarthy, J. W., & Smith, J. L. (2012). Situational and psychosocial factors mediating coordinated joint attention with augmentative and alternative communication systems with beginning communicators without disabilities. *Augmentative and Alternative Communication, 27*(2), 67–76.

Bornstein, M. H., & Tamis-LeMonda, C. S. (2010). Parent-infant interaction. In *The Wiley-Blackwell handbook of infant development* (pp. 458–482). West Sussex, UK: Wiley-Blackwell.

Braddock, B., McDaniel, J., Spragge, S., Loncke, F., Braddock, S. R., & Carey, J. C. (2012). Communication ability in persons with trisomy 18 and trisomy 13. *Augmentative and Alternative Communication, 28*(4), 266–277.

Braddock, B., Pickett, C., Ezzelgot, J., Sheth, S., Korte-Stroff, E., Loncke, F., & Block, L. (2013). Potential communicative acts in children with autism spectrum disorders. *Developmental Neurorehabilitation.*

Branson, D., & Demchak, M. (2009). The use of augmentative and alternative communication methods with infants and toddlers with disabilities: A research review. *Augmentative and Alternative Communication, 25*(4), 274–286.

Brown, R. W. (1973). *A first language; The early stages.* Cambridge, MA: Harvard University Press.

Capirci, O., Iverson, J. M., Pizzuto, E., & Volterra, V. (1996). Gestures and words during the transition to two-word speech. *Journal of Child Language, 23*(3), 645–673.

Clark, E. V. (2009). *First language acquisition* (2nd ed.). New York, NY: Cambridge University Press.

Cress, C. J., & Marvin, C. A. (2003). Common questions about AAC services in early intervention. *Augmentative and Alternative Communication, 19*(4), 254–272.

Fenson, L., Marchman, V. A., Thal, D., Dale, P., Reznick, J., & Bates, E. (2007). *The MacArthur-Bates communicative development inventories: User's guide and technical manual* (2nd ed.). Baltimore, MD: Paul H. Brookes.

Fiske, S. (2010). *Social beings: Core motives in social psychology.* New York, NY: Wiley.

Gaskell, M. G., & Ellis, A. W. (2009). Word learning and lexical development across the lifespan. *Philosophical Transactions of the Royal Society of Biological Sciences, 364*(1536), 3607–3615.

Gillette, Y. (2003). *Achieving communication independence. A comprehensive guide to assessment and intervention for persons with severe communication disabilities and AAC users.* Eau Claire, WI: Thinking Publications.

Goldin-Meadow, S. (2009). From gesture to word. In E. Bavin (Ed.), *The Cambridge handbook of child language* (pp. 145–160). Cambridge, UK: Cambridge University Press.

Harley, T. A. (2008). *The psychology of language: From data to theory* (3rd ed.). New York, NY: Psychology Press.

Kangas, K. A., & Lloyd, L. L. (1988). Early cognitive skills as prerequisites to augmentative and alternative communication use: What are we waiting for? *Augmentative and Alternative Communication, 4*(4), 211.

Olsson, C., & Granlund, M. (2003). Communication intervention for pre-symbolic communication. In R. W. Schlosser (Ed.). *Efficacy research in augmentative and alternative communication.* New York, NY: Elsevier.

Piaget, J. (1974, 1926). *The language and thought of the child* (trans. M. Gabain). New York, NY: New American Library. [*Le langage et la pensée chez l'enfant.* Neuchatel, Switzerland: Delachaux et Niestle.]

Reed, G. M., Lux, J. B., Bufka, L. F., Trask, C., Peterson, D. B., Stark, S., & Hawley, J. A. (2005). Operationalizing the International Classification of Functioning, Disability and Health in clinical settings. *Rehabilitation Psychology, 50*(2), 122–131.

Reichle, J., & Wacker, D. (Eds.). (1993). *Communicative alternatives to challenging behavior. Integrating functional assessment and intervention strategies.* Baltimore, MD: Paul H. Brookes.

Repp, A. C., & Horner, R. H. (Eds.). (1999). *Functional analysis of problem behavior. From effective assessment to effective support.* Belmont, CA: Wadsworth.

Romski, M., & Sevcik, R. A. (2005). Augmentative communication and early intervention: Myths and realities. *Infants and Young Children, 18*(3), 174–185.

Siegel, E., & Wetherby, A. (2006). Nonsymbolic communication. In M. E. Snell, & F. Brown (Eds.), *Instruction of students with severe disabilities* (6th ed., pp. 405–446). Upper Saddle River, NJ: Merrill.

Sigafoos, J., Drasgow, E., & Schlosser, R. (2003). Strategies for beginning communicators. In R. Schlosser (Ed.), *The efficacy of augmentative and alternative communication* (pp. 323–346). New York, NY: Elsevier.

Sigafoos, J., & Mirenda, P. (2002). Strengthening communicative behaviors for gaining access to desired items and activities. In J. Reichle, D. R. Beukelman, & J. Light (Eds.), *Exemplary practices for beginning communicators: Implications for AAC* (pp. 123–156). Baltimore, MD: Paul H. Brookes.

Sigafoos, J., Woodyatt, G., Deen, D., Tait, K., Tucker, M., Roberts-Pennell, D., & Pittendreigh, N. (2000). Identifying potential communicative acts in children with developmental and physical disabilities. *Communication Disorders Quarterly, 21*, 77–86.

Snell, M. (2002). Using dynamic assessment with learners who communicate nonsymbolically. *Augmentative and Alternative Communication, 18*(3), 163–176.

Snell, M. E., Berlin, R. A., Voorhees, M. D., Stanton-Chapman, T. L., & Hadden, S. (2012). A survey of preschool staff concerning problem behavior and its prevention in Head Start classrooms. *Journal of Positive Behavior Interventions, 14*(2), 98–107.

Snell, M., & Loncke, F. (2002, 2005). *Manual for the dynamic assessment of nonsymbolic communication* [Translated into Spanish by the Department of Participation and Solidarity in Education in Andalucia, Motril/Granada, Spain] (Unpublished manuscript).

Tomasello, M. (1988). The role of joint attentional processes in early language development. *Language Sciences, 10*(1), 69–88.

Tomasello, M. (2008). *Origins of human communication.* Cambridge, MA: MIT Press.

Tomasello, M. (2009). The usage-based theory of language acquisition. In E. Bavin (Ed.), *The Cambridge handbook of child language* (pp. 69–87). Cambridge, UK: Cambridge University Press.

Virginia Department of Education Office of Special Education and Student Services. (2011). *Speech-language pathology services in schools: Guidelines for best practice*. Richmond, VA: Author.

Walker, V. L., & Snell, M. E. (2013). Effects of augmentative and alternative communication on challenging behavior: A meta-analysis. *Augmentative and Alternative Communication, 29*(2), 117–131.

Watzlawick, P., Bavelas, J. B., & Jackson, D. D. (1967). *Pragmatics of human communication; A study of interactional patterns, pathologies, and paradoxes*. New York, NY: Norton.

Wetherby, A., & Prizant, B. (1989). The expression of communicative intent: Assessment issues. *Seminars in Speech & Language, 10,* 77–91.

Wetherby, A. M., & Prizant, B. M. (2002). *Communication and symbolic behavior scales: Developmental profile* (1st ed.). Baltimore, MD: Paul H. Brookes.

CHAPTER 7

Language Intervention and AAC

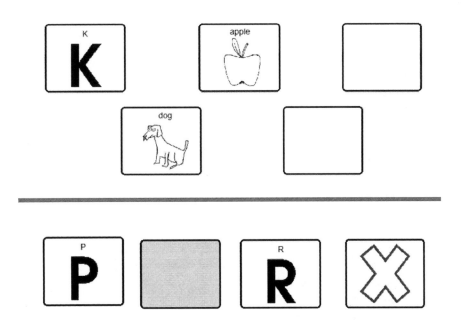

Is the purpose of AAC the facilitation of communication, or the facilitation of acquisition and use of language? Or both? Of course, this depends on age, educational goals, developmental abilities, and other factors. It is clear that language goals can be highly desirable for children and adolescents and also for individuals with acquired linguistic disorders (aphasia) who may recover the use of language.

This chapter explores how the use of AAC affects a person's acquisition, knowledge, mastery, and use of language. One of the most salient characteristics of AAC is the fact that in many of its appli-cations, a modality other than natural speech is used for expression. What is the relation between the externally observable mode of expression (natural speech, manual signing, device-generated speech, graphic symbols) and language, which is an internalized system? Is the language system of a person who uses manual signs different than that of a person who uses natural speech? Does the user of manual signs develop internalized phonological representations? Will a person who uses key word signing (the use of signs for the words of an utterance that carry most of the meaning) internally develop a simplified, telegraphic syntax? And what about people who use graphic symbols? Do they develop an internal visual symbol grammar that is different from the grammar of the spoken language?

From a theoretical point of view, these questions are fascinating. If research can focus on these and similar questions, we could obtain answers about the interaction between modality and system. AAC research could help us to disentangle problems such as: which one came first, speech or language? Are our language characteristics adapted to what natural speech allows us to do? If so, is that the reason why natural sign languages used by communities of deaf people would have their own characteristics?

The study of AAC could have the potential to provide clues into the relation between internal language characteristics and the modality of expression. By observing how individuals learn, converse, and strategize with AAC in order to build and deconstruct messages out of symbols, manual signs with different speed and other nonsymbolic forms, we may learn something about how language adapts itself to varying conditions.

Let us focus first on the questions that need to be asked, and explore how AAC might provide an answer (Loncke, 2008):

1. How are the main mechanisms of language acquisition affected by the use of AAC?
2. What is the effect of the decreased output possibilities?
3. What do we know about the developing lexicon?
4. What do we know about: (1) phonology, (2) morphology, and (3) syntax development?
5. How does the use of AAC affect literacy?

6. Are there specific language stimulating strategies that can be adopted by clinicians and educators?

These questions explore the hypothesis that the use of AAC creates a different acquisition and functioning environment for the person.

1. How Are the Main Mechanisms of Language Acquisition Affected by the Use of AAC?

Although there are major debates about how much of language acquisition can be attributed to an innate component and how much is the result of learning from environmental experience, there is general agreement that language acquisition is made possible through a convergence of: (1) biological factors, (2) language exposure, (3) cognitive challenges, and (4) social regulators.

Biological Factors

Biological factors include the genetic constitution of the person, the physiological and anatomical structures, and the wiring and functioning of the central nervous system. It should be remembered that, in many cases, individuals who will potentially rely on AAC may have deficiencies or dysfunctions that are either congenital or acquired at a later developmental or life state. Although this certainly may limit the scope of the objectives that will be reached through intervention, it does not take away the fact that individuals possess a large degree of learning and acquisition potential. It is essential to understand and further explore the genetic and medical diagnoses and how these translate into expectations for clinical and educational rehabilitation and intervention.

Language Exposure

How can we characterize the *language* that AAC users (or AAC candidates) are *exposed* to? While there is no reason to expect that there is anything inherent in the condition of AAC use that would alter the language used directed to the user, AAC users will likely receive less language input as a direct result of their own decreased communicative expressions (Grove & Smith, 1997). The more you speak, the more you receive responses. Compared with typical communicators, AAC users will most likely be talked to less frequently. However, this is not simply because they talk less. Another factor that plays into it is that communication partners somehow realize that interaction with an AAC user will require more effort, more concentration, and more time. Talking with an AAC user or an AAC candidate is usually not as effortless as typical communication. Introducing AAC is aimed to counter this phenomenon: by giving the persons a way to express themselves, ask questions, make comments, and socialize in many ways, one aims at reversing the downward spiral of lack of linguistic exposure and expectations. To prevent such a downward spiral, it is essential to introduce AAC as early in the development of the child as possible: make communication effective and raise the expectations in caregivers and all communication partners.

Cognitive Challenges

Language is a cognitive tool that allows the user to label information and use structures to examine and express how things relate, how events unfold, and how they are grasped in thoughts (Tomasello, 2003). As children acquire language and extend their lexicon, they use it as a mental organizational internalized tool that helps their thinking, mental planning, and emotional cognitive behavior. At this point, it is an understudied aspect within AAC research how much the introduction of AAC does or can contribute to cognitive growth.

Social Regulations

Language use is steered by social feedback. Children and adolescents learn such functions as naming, questioning, answering, comparing, and discussing, through interactive operations in which communication partners (peers, siblings, as well as parents) reinforce, correct, and recast language use. The countless interactions help children to build pragmatic linguistic skills that allow them to become successful linguistic participants. All this is not so evident for AAC users who seldom can observe other pragmatically competent AAC users. Parents and caregivers need to pay special attention to this need (Todman & Alm, 2003).

2. What Is the Effect of the Decreased Output Possibilities?

Each time a child or an adult speaks, they hear themselves talk, which provides an autofeedback. Often communication partners will respond or react to their utterances, what can be called external feedback. This feedback to one's own expression provides a basic for learning and verbal practice.

When young children use words, it becomes clear that they are exploring the semantic specifics and the semantic range of the words. They may initially think that "daddy" stands for any adult male, until they figure out that "daddy" and "man" are two different words, be it that they have some semantic traits in common (human beings, males, adults). This is an example of overextension (together with its counterpart underextension, for example thinking that the word "cat" only applies to the one in your home). It shows how by actively using words and observing their environment's reaction (external feedback) (sometimes a correction, sometimes laughter, occasionally embarrassment), children figure out really fast what words mean. Developmental psychologists describe the so-called vocabulary spurt as a period between the ages of 2 and 5 during which normally developing children show an amazing ability to produce speech after minimal exposure. In short, children learn well and amazingly fast if they can actively (i.e., through using the words in real contexts) try out hundreds of words every day. It is easy to realize that this is something for which young users of AAC are in a less favorable situation, for the reasons that have been discussed in other chapters: (1) AAC users simply may "have" less words (as they need to be on their boards or their devices—or, in case of manual signs, they need to be explicitly "taught"), and (2) producing the words requires much more effort for AAC users (because of physical access limitations, and—often—the need to go through an external device as an intermediary to produce the words, which requires a specific kind of operational competence).

Grove and Smith (1997) call this the problem of *asymmetry* between input and output. Children who are AAC users contribute extremely little to conversations because of a combination of factors such as: (1) fewer words and messages are available, (2) accessing the words requires much more effort and time, (3) the difficulty to keep up with the pace of the conversation (when you are ready to make your comment, the conversation has already moved on to the next topic, and you look and sound foolish if you still make your comment), and (4) the chance that communication partners lower their expectations (they may not even ask questions or include the person in the conversation as they have the experience that responses maybe slow, hard to understand, and confusing).

Soto and Toro-Zambrana (1995) found that users of Bliss symbols sometimes used syntactic combinations that appeared to be idiosyncratic. However, upon nearer inspection, they discovered that these idiosyncratic symbol sequences were rule-governed and were "visually" meaningful. Hoag, Bedrosian, and McCoy (2004) describe the trade-off between informativeness and speed when AAC users deliver messages. In a controlled natural environment, the authors observed which strategies AAC users employed when they had to convey explicit information in a natural situation (e.g., talking to a clerk at a check-out counter). Although there are a range of individual and situational differences between how effective the communication is, it is clear that all AAC users seem to strike some form of compromise between how much information to give, how to structure it (structurally- linguistically), and how fast the message can or must be delivered. From a pragmatic-functional point of view, the grammaticality of the utterance does not seem to be a major concern of the AAC users. They need to get their message across and fast (and effectively). Maybe grammaticality is really never much of a concern for language users. Maybe individuals are simply driven by the desire to be explicit and clear—to make communication work and be effective—and typical speakers use grammar simply because it is there and it comes so easily. In other words, grammar works as a tool for quickly structuring what you have to say. But it will be dropped as a tool (and replaced by something else) if it doesn't do the job. This could be one of the areas where AAC can provide us with interesting data to test hypotheses about general human cognition!

Taken all together, AAC is an important push toward communication for individuals who have limited access to the typical forms of language (natural speech, writing). On the one hand, this increases the person's chances to acquire and learn language. The more you communicate in language, the better you get at it. However, on the other hand, the very nature of the modalities used in AAC and the speed issue may drive the individual away from the grammatical forms used in typical language. Therefore, the challenge for educators is to maximize communication (and remember: grammar-poor communication is much better than no communication!) while at the same time doing everything one can to allow language development and language acquisition. A challenge for language educators and speech-language pathologists.

3. What Do We Know About the Developing Lexicon?

The problem of the developing lexicon has been discussed in Chapter 5. The essence is that AAC users are often highly dependent on the words (the selection of words and the number of words) that the caregivers make available to them. Caregivers often assume a limited-word-learning-

capacity and therefore let the lexicon only grow slowly and in a planned way. That is certainly not what happens in typical nondisabled language users. The vocabulary spurt, well described in language acquisition literature, might simply never happen if the lexical development would be subject to planning by educators, assuming a limited word learning capacity.

Educators and speech-language pathologists may hesitate to "unleash" an unlimited lexicon on the AAC user. An educationally workable method might be to make a distinction between "targeted words," of which the active use will be part of the learning objectives, and the "wealth of words" that will be used and made available to the child to use freely. The problem with providing a wealth of words to AAC users is no longer that devices would not have the capacity to hold the words and phrases, but that the user needs to acquire navigating or coding (e.g., in semantic compaction) strategies that take time and could put an enormous burden on the speaker (and the listener).

However, do we really need to strive for a lexicon that is maximally extended? For some of the AAC users, maybe less would be better? Individuals with limited cognitive linguistic potential might indeed benefit from a more limited lexicon. If chosen well, a limited lexicon that contains words that can be used in multiple contexts (words as such as "why," "yes," "I," "give," etc.) might be preferable over thousands of words—forcing the person to "manage" a huge lexicon.

Managing the lexicon for an AAC user requires a different set of skills than those that are needed by nondisabled speakers to manage their mental lexicons. Users of speech-generating devices need to literally "find their way" (i.e., navigate) to and through the lexicon. Again, the study of AAC use may help us to investigate some of the more general cognitive-linguistic problems. Take the old question how many words language users have. Do normal nondisabled adult speakers "know" 50,000 words? Or is it rather 70,000? Or is it more? All these numbers are out there. The problem is that the question is unanswerable as long as we don't know exactly how the internal mental system deals with words. Is *possible, impossible, possibility, impossibility,* just one word with different additions, or are these four different words separately stored in your mind? In other words, do we know these four words, or do we know one single word with different variations according to semantically specific requirements?

This brings us to the question of what should be the goals of language therapy for AAC users? Should we focus on identifying and finding all the words, or should we focus more on strategies to "assemble" the words based on knowledge of codes? The limitations of AAC for lexical access (slow speed, restricted lexicon) are the source of a debate of the use of fringe and core vocabulary, how to best program pages within a device, and the pros and cons of a specially designed system of combinatorial syntax for AAC like icon sequencing (Hill & Spurk, 2004).

4. What Do We Know About: (1) Phonology, (2) Morphology, and (3) Syntax Development?

Phonology is the first linguistic component to develop fully in normally developing children. As the lack of functional speech is the main characteristic of almost all the candidates and users of AAC, one can expect that the development of pho-

nology will be weak. In typical development, the phenomenon and stage of babbling (starting around the age of 6–8 months) is largely seen as a natural stage in which children practice speech output and match it with the phonological repertoire that they perceive in their environment. Most children who will need to rely on AAC do not babble and cannot benefit from these spontaneous psychomotor exercices.

In how far do AAC users actually develop an internal phonological component? In a series of studies, Loncke and associates (Loncke, Hilton, Weng, & Corthals, 2009) attempted to measure whether the presence of speech output in AAC could be beneficial for the development of internalized phonological representations. They asked nondisabled college students to learn and try to remember pseudowords that had been associated with varying combinations of: (1) sound output (they heard the pseudo-word produced by a computer or a speech-generating device), (2) an iconic manual sign, (3) a noniconic manual sign, and (4) an orthographic representation. The underlying reasoning was that the mental storage of words is strengthened by associated stimuli and that it would be interesting to know which of the added modalities (the speech output, the manual sign) would have the stronger effect on learning. The results indicated that words with a simple phonological structure (e.g., "lafid") do not need to have extra support form other modalities—the participants did fine regardless which combination of modalities that was added to the stimuli. However, when more complex words needed to be learned and memorized (e.g, "kominalzur"), added modalities did play a beneficial role, such as auditory input (from the speech generating device or the computer), which helped to remember. Simple words ("lafid") are easily stored and remembered. Here is one possible explanation: the auditory input helps to create an internalized phonological schema that helps the user in storing and accessing the information. Does this also apply to AAC users? Although there is little direct research, psycholinguistic evidence does indeed suggest that an internal phonological representation helps in accessing and internally structuring words. If this is the case, then the use of speech-generating devices is not only beneficial for direct communication; it helps the user to build an internal phonology.

Morphology and Syntax

In typical English acquisition, morphology and syntax are often considered to be the most difficult components to fully acquire and master (Blackwell & Bates, 1995). One reason for this phenomenon might be that utterances with morphological deficiencies may still be communicatively effective. Another factor that may play a role is the effort-outcome trade-off. Focusing on morphology and word agreement may require relatively hard work from typical children in stages at which their communication is relatively effective without morphology. This can be even more the case for individuals who use AAC—adding morphological markers to lexical stems does not only require cognitive-linguistic effort, but also important memory and physical effort. Considering the fact that speed of utterance generation is a crucial element in communication effectiveness, morphology may strategically be a low priority for the language user. This is comparable with observations and studies of the use of text messaging, instant messaging,

and e-mailing, where high occurrence of abbreviations and morphological neglect have been reported in otherwise typical language users (Ling & Baron, 2007).

5. How Does the Use of AAC Affect Literacy?

Or maybe the first question should be: how does the nonuse of AAC affect literacy? (see also Chapter 9). The need for AAC comes from the fact that the person does not have (or cannot develop) functional speech. This can be caused by a range of factors (e.g., neuromotor in case of cerebral palsy, or neurogenetic in case of some forms of autism) that can directly have an effect on limitations in the ability to learn to read and write (see Chapter 9). Here we suffice with mentioning that AAC users are at risk for impaired literacy development because of the nature of language and communication in which they participate: (1) AAC users are more likely to have significantly less language and communicative experience—both in terms of language to which they are exposed and language they can actively use; and (2) Educators tend not to have the same expectations of AAC users as they have of typical speakers. AAC existed for several years as a subdiscipline within special education, speech-language pathology, and rehabilitations sciences before there was any emerging interest for literacy. I would say that this is understandable, as AAC rose as an applied subdiscipline to "give a voice" to people who couldn't speak. Initially, the main goal was to find a way out of the limitations of being isolated—direct communication from person-to-person was (and is) understandably the first concern. The focus on literacy, therefore, came later.

LANGUAGE LEARNING THROUGH INTERACTION

Parents (and others) who communicate with children who are AAC users need to adopt adapted rules of interacting. These are needed to increase the language learning benefits of the interaction. Light, McNaughton, and Parnes (1986) and Jonker and Heim (1992) and Heim (2010) discuss a series of "partner strategies" that can be used to make parents (and others) aware of how their interactive behavior can be a facilitator (or, if not used appropriately, a hindrance) for communicative learning. These "partner strategies" include:

1. *Structure the environment.* Make sure you are in the visual field of the child. Position yourself at eye-height of the child. Remove visual and auditory detractors;

2. *Follow the child's lead.* Avoid being the dominant force in setting the topic of the conversation. It requires skill and self-discipline to give time to the child to indicate what his or her contribution to the conversation is. It is important to give the child a role in topic-setting. In many cases, the child will indicate in a nonverbal way what they want or what they desire to comment about. Because nonverbal messages often contain a large amount of ambiguity, one needs to be cautious not to over-interpret or misinterpret the message;

3. *Solicit a shared focus.* Already during the very first year in development, caregivers of typically developing children seem to have the sensitivity to detect what it is that is of interest to the baby. Parents will use this to

comment to the baby, and they will be encouraged when the baby smiles or shows signs of response. Studies have revealed that parents of children with cerebral palsy have much more difficulty in establishing joint contact and interest, for the simple reason that functions such as visual focusing and attention may be disturbed. Furthermore, the child's behavior and intentions are often harder to interpret by the parents because of involuntary movements and motor coordination problems. Communication partners of children with cerebral palsy (or other severe developmental disorders) need to be instructed to actively seek joint attention and not be discouraged by signals that can be interpreted as inattention;

4. *Provide opportunities for communicative interaction.* People talk about their needs (what they like and what they don't like) and comment on everything they find of interest (and that they suspect their communication partners will find interesting). Communication partners should look for and use topics and events that present themselves and that may capture the child's attention;

5. *Expect communication/interaction that is appropriate for the child.* Individuals who are developmentally delayed may show characteristics of a child younger than their own age. However, at the same time they may have interests that are perfectly in line with what you would expect of a person of their age. A 14-year-old girl is likely to show some of the behaviors that are typical for teenagers, even if at some moments her behavior may remind you more of an 8-year-old. We

should be careful to avoid infantilizing behavior on our part (e.g., talking to a teenager as if she is a toddler);

6. *Pace the interaction (Pause).* Nondisabled communicators tend to feel the need to "say something" while they are waiting for the person's response. Doing this, a second conversation gets superimposed over the ongoing conversation, and it further strengthens the dominance of the nondisabled communicator;

7. *Provide models for the modes within the child's repertoire.* Most AAC users seldom (or never) see other AAC users. How are they supposed to figure out how it is done? Therefore, it is important that the communication partners themselves also use the communication device in an interaction. This should be even easier for the use of nontech communication systems (boards, and certainly the use of manual signs). If manual signing is done by all caregivers, it becomes a "normal" behavior, and as a result, it will be more likely adopted by the AAC user.

The sociolinguistic phenomenon of "code-switching" is another reason why modeling is important. Code-switching refers to the tendency that individuals seek linguistic conformity. You detect what language is "right" or "appropriate" for a given situation (i.e., one tends to speak/communicate the way others in the group do). Many people have different speaking styles at home and at the office, and automatically switch to the appropriate style when they enter a situation. A bilingual French-English speaker will automatically switch from English to French depending on the situation (i.e., on the language that

is spoken in the environment). But that same speaker will find it awkward when asked to speak French in an English environment (or English in a French environment). If you apply this principle to AAC users, then it is no longer a surprise that there is AAC abandonment. As an AAC user, you find yourself constantly violating the linguistic conformity rule! One partial solution for this problem may be to make the communication partners use some of the AAC tools too. In other words, you may want to try to make AAC less exceptional (most people don't want to be the exception) and more normal (you make the AAC way of communicating the norm).

8. *Provide appropriate language input.* Parents of young typically developing children often sense exactly how much their child understands. Intuitively, these parents adapt their style of communication to what can be processed by the child. Children with cerebral palsy are "harder to read" by their parents. Nevertheless, by asking questions or by asking the child to respond to requests, one can often (in a dynamic assessment way, see also Chapter 11) determine the range of what is within reach of the child's comprehension. Use language, gestures, and objects that are likely to be understood by the child;

9. *Prompt.* Good partner behavior includes encouragement for the child to respond or otherwise contribute to the conversation. Partners indicate through verbal and nonverbal signals that they expect something from the child. For example, communication partners who feel insecure or who

do not expect that the child has the capacity or the desire to communicate will—in most cases unconsciously—indicate just that to the child;

10. *Reward all communicative attempts.* Partners who respond to all communicative attempts will increase the child's confidence and desire to participate. It should be remembered that passivity is enemy number one for individuals who rely on AAC. Unfortunately, many well-meaning caregivers reinforce passivity by not noticing and honoring the child's communicative attempts.

LANGUAGE USE WITH AAC

There are some indications that children who are AAC users might produce language utterances that do not match the syntactic level of their non-AAC using peers. Let us take a look at some of the data.

Grove and Dockrell (2000) studied the spontaneous utterances of children with intellectual disabilities who were using manual signing. They found that the utterances only rarely exceed the one-sign or two-sign structure. Is this an indication that they were limited in their linguistic development? Interestingly, there were a number of utterances that were clearly not a direct transposition of the structure of a spoken sentence. The authors wonder if these hearing children with intellectual disabilities were exploring the possibilities of a visual-manual grammatical structure. This is an interesting idea: Would the medium of AAC lend itself to structures that are different from the spoken language? At present, there is a wealth of sign language linguistic research that indicate

that some of the grammatical features of sign languages are influenced by the need to process information in the visual-simultaneous way (as opposed to the auditory-successive processing of spoken language; Valli, Lucas, & Mulrooney, 2005).

Blockberger and Johnston (2003) compared three groups of children on a number of language tasks: children with extremely limited speech, children with typical speech but delayed language development, and typically developing children. The children with severe limitations in natural speech performed with markedly more difficulty than the other two groups in such tasks as comprehension and morphological judgment. As can be expected, the more difficulty you have in producing speech during the time of acquisition, the more it will threaten your ability to acquire the grammar of the language in its entirety. In other words, acquisition of language is highly dependent on practice! Here is where AAC comes in: a communication method (unaided or aided) is not only beneficial because it lets the person interact with the environment. In doing so, one leans the rules of the code (the language) that is underlying the communication.

But is the use of the communication system really teaching you the language? Could it be that users of devices or other AAC methods are actually learning a code that is different from standard language? Could it be that the communication means that we give through AAC guides them to different structures? We know that the structure of sign languages is different from that of spoken language, probably because the syntax is based on a "visual" organization of information. Instead of the typical "English" subject-verb-object preferential structure, many sign languages tend to prefer a subject-object-verb structure. Most sign languages would favor the order I-you-hate to express "I hate you." Why? The most probable explanation is that in a visual representation, you will need to bring up the players first before you can indicate what the action between the two actors consists of. Interestingly, this could explain some of the results of the Grove and Dockrell (2000) study that we mentioned earlier. Several of the hearing children with developmental delays who were exposed to manual signing showed what they called "nonconventional patterns" where one could easily see that the utterance was not a transposition of English. In some of the utterances, the information was indeed handled in ways similar to that of a young deaf child growing up in a sign language-using environment would use.

Sutton and Morford (1998) looked at the constituent order in picture pointing sequences by speaking children. Younger children obviously are not yet guided by the structure of the spoken language when they successively point to pictures to indicate "who is doing what to whom." Thus, it could be that it is the "visual" nature of utterance construction that invites the user to come up with different structures. In another study, Sutton et al. (2002) wanted to know how 3- to 4-year-old children would construct messages with pictures. The results show that the children are not merely transposing their language skills to a graphic representation. Again, it is the visual-spatial nature of the pictures that guides how they construct a relationship between the elements.

There is obviously some uncertainty about what it means to use an alternative mode of communication for the acquisition of the typical language structures. However, this does not mean that thera-pists cannot use the communication device to advance linguistic mastery of English (or the spoken language used by the child's environment). Binger and Light (2007) explored the possibilities of aided AAC modeling. Working with preschoolers who used communication devices, they set up a training consisting of pointing to symbols and symbol combinations on the device and providing a complete spoken model. Four of the five children showed the ability to generalize, which had long-term learning effects. These authors obviously hit on something basic that is easily forgotten: that it will not be sufficient to hand the communication device over to children and expect that they will spontaneously start generating English sentences. Without external structuring, it is quite possible that the child will simply make "sensible combinations" that are not necessarily congruent with well-formed English sentences.

AMOUNT OF EXPOSURE TO COMMUNICATION AND ITS INFLUENCE

What do people communicate about? People talk about their lives. They talk about what drives them, what fascinates them, and what challenges them cognitively. The more a person lives in a predictable world, the less there is a need to communicate. The more a person lives in a world that offers new experiences, the more there will be a need to speak, to ask questions, to comment, to protest, and to discuss. Individuals who use or need AAC often live and function in predictable and repetitive world with similar sequences of events, and hence with fewer needs and expectations to communicate. Experience, cognitive challenges, and communicative expressions feed into each other constantly. An increase of experience and challenges leads to more experiences and more challenges, leading to more communication. Conversely, a decrease of experience and challenges shrinks the potential of cognitive exploration and decreases the need to communicate.

Decreased communication leads to decreased *social participation*. Everywhere, individuals work and function together and will implement *negotiating, consensus seeking, debating, protesting, schmoozing, threatening, convincing, seducing,* and more pragmatic functions. Social participation allows you to learn the "skills of the whole scope of pragmatics" and improve as you practice and gain more experience. Less social participation—and that is where many AAC users and AAC candidates find themselves—will give you less opportunity to learn these pragmatic-linguistic functions. This is not the only reason why some AAC users may occasionally display pragmatic awkwardness. One other important reason is that they often lack models of "how you get things done if you are an AAC user"?

Pragmatics—getting things done—is very much about getting the timing right for speaking and also pulling in the right nonverbal ingredients. The right word at the right time with the right kind of smile (or serious face) can do it—but that will differ if a person is in a wheelchair using an AAC device! This is one reason why it is important for AAC users to spend time together (e.g., during a camp) and be able to observe each other (observational learning). This, quite naturally, will have an impact on the acquisition of language skills.

LEARNING STRUCTURES AND STRATEGIES

This brings us to the learning processes that we would like to encourage through therapeutic sessions and, maybe even more importantly, through daily interaction.

Modeling

Modeling is certainly an important factor in learning structures—and perhaps the best way of modeling is when the communication partner (the clinician) uses the device (or the AAC modality). It is also powerful if peers could be included in this learning process. It is proven that modeling works better if the learner identifies with the model—teenagers may rather identify with their peers than with a boring clinician! Other general principles used in almost all forms of language therapy should be applicable as well.

Recasting

In typical development, parents quite naturally provide children with responses to their linguistic utterances that reinforce newly produced structures or help them discover new syntactic and expanded syntactic structures. This phenomenon, called linguistic recasting is often assumed to be a central mechanism that promotes language acquisition. For example, parents would, quite naturally, respond to a child's utterance "Car fast" with something like, "Yes, the car is fast. It is a fast car." But does this principle also apply to AAC use? Several authors believe that AAC recasting is or should be, indeed, a central principle in the intervention. Recasting is believed to be a powerful mechanism that helps the children to cognitively compare their own utterances with an "improved" version provided by the adult. The adult provides contrasting information, which allows the child to focus on the "missing element" (or the element that needs to be corrected; Nelson, 1989). It is supposed to help the child proceed to a higher, more advanced level of grammatical construction and comprehension. Fey (2008) argues that the recasting principle should be a guiding directive for improving language output in AAC users. Would recasting be something that needs to be practiced more and systematically in interaction with children who use AAC? Would that provide an impetus that will allow them to develop and acquire language faster?

Essentially, recasting is a response by the communication partner that contains the same information that the child has given in his/her utterance plus added structural information (sometimes a grammatical correction) or content. For example, in response to the child's utterance, "Paul run," the adult would respond, "Yes, Paul will run" (according to the context). What happens in the child's head when you recast such as used in this example? You hope that the child will make a cognitive comparison between the new structure (Paul will run) and the current structure (i.e., the child's own structure: Paul run). Nelson (1989) suggests that there are three possibilities—(1) the child simply doesn't notice the differences between the structures. Nelson (1989) and many others suggest that this is what happens most of the time. Most frequently, our recasts and comments go "in one ear, out the other ear," but sometimes—when the right mixture of motivation, attention, and linguistic readiness are there (Nelson talks about the "tricky mix"), the child does

grab the information and notice the added information, (2) the child does notice that what the clinician says is "different" than what he or she said themselves, but the child is unable to further process or analyze this information, or (3) the child does notice a "codable" difference. "Codable" here means that the child sees through the structure of the new utterance and is able to copy the new structure.

Another strategy borrowed from language therapy principles is the use of *social scripting.* The use of repetitive (with variations) sequences of information exchange through activities such as book reading, meal preparation, meal time, thematic play ("house," "space," etc.), and visiting other families, can contribute to the child's successful attention to and analysis of new forms.

Are these principles usable and should they be used in language therapy (and general language activities) with children who use AAC? Absolutely! Talk to language teachers about this—they can do a lot of fun stuff that is language stimulating. For too long, the focus has been on providing the AAC users with means that allow them to express what they have to say, and we have not paid enough attention to the enormous possibilities of AAC for (structural) language development. There is no law against recasting with an AAC device! In therapy sessions, speech-language pathologists should have parts of their sessions mainly establishing a conversational exchange that will allow the clinician to provide structural feedback through recasting. The use of social scripts may be even more promising. One can program the communication device with messages, comments, instructions that go with the script (in fact, you could enter the entire script in the communication device). And why not throw in some funny comments? A great way of exploring pragmatics! Book reading and AAC is almost a chapter on its own! There is a whole body of literature that underscores the importance of book reading for children's literacy development (Cunningham & Stanovich, 1998). This is no less important for children who are AAC users.

POINTS TO REMEMBER

- AAC can be used to improve communication, language, and cognition. Communicative goals (effective exchange of signals) are not always linguistic in nature or may favor a different structure.
- Acquiring and developing language as an AAC user may be dramatically different from typical language learners because of decreased input, different message management requirements, and a communicatively asymmetrical relation with non-AAC using partners.
- Language performance in AAC may be characterized by nontypical use of morphology, and order of elements. This does not necessarily indicate a language disorder, but may be caused by message management requirements such as speed.
- Language therapeutic principles such as recasting are applicable to AAC users if language performance is a goal of the intervention.

REFERENCES

Binger, C., & Light, J. (2007). The effect of aided AAC modeling on the expression of multi-symbol messages by preschoolers who use AAC. *AAC: Augmentative and Alternative Communication, 23*(1), 30–43.

Blackwell, A., & Bates, E. (1995). Inducing agrammatic profiles in normals: Evidence for the selective vulnerability of morphology under cognitive resource limitation. *Journal of Cognitive Neuroscience, 7*(2), 228–257.

Blockberger, S., & Johnston, J. R. (2003). Grammatical morphology acquisition by children with complex communication needs. *AAC: Augmentative and Alternative Communication, 19*(4), 207–221.

Cunningham, A. E., & Stanovich, K. E. (1998). What reading does for the mind. *American Educator*, pp. 8–15.

Fey, M. E. (2008). Thoughts on grammar intervention in AAC. *Perspectives in Augmentative Communication. American Speech-Language and Hearing Association. The Division 12 Newsletter.*

Grove, N., & Dockrell, J. (2000). Multisign combinations by children with intellectual impairments: An analysis of language skills. *Journal of Speech, Language, and Hearing Research, 43*(2), 309–323.

Grove, N., & Smith, M. (1997). Input-output asymmetry: Language development in augmentative and alternative communication. *ISAAC Bulletin, 5*, 1–3.

Heim, M. (2010). *Effects of the COCP program in children and youngsters with profound intellectual and multiple disabilities.* 14th Biennial Conference of the International Society for Augmentative and Alternative Communication, Barcelona, Spain.

Hill, K., & Spurk, E. (2004). AAC performance based on semantic organization schemes using dynamic displays. *Proceedings of the 2004 RESNA Annual Conference* [CD-ROM].

Hoag, L. A., Bedrosian, J. L., & McCoy, K. F. (2004). Trade-offs between informativeness and speed of message delivery in augmentative and alternative communication. *Journal of Speech, Language, and Hearing Research, 47*(6), 1270–1285.

Jonker, V., & Heim, M. (1992). *A communication program for non-speaking children and their partners* (unpublished manuscript). Paper presented at the Biennial International Conference of the International Society for Augmentative and Alternative Communication, Philadelphia, PA.

Light, J., McNaughton, D., & Parnes, P. (1986). *A protocol for the assessment of the communicative interaction skills of nonspeaking severely handi-capped adults and their facilitators.* Toronto, Canada: Augmentative Communication Service, Hugh MacMillan Medical Centre.

Ling, R., & Baron, N. S. (2007). Text messaging and IM: Linguistic comparison of American College data. *Journal of Language and Social Psychology, 26*(3), 291–298.

Loncke, F. (2008). Basic principles of language intervention in children who use AAC. *Perspectives on Augmentative and Alternative Communication, 17*, 50–55.

Loncke, F., Hilton, J., Weng, P., & Corthals, P. (2009). *Testing the multimodality hypothesis. learning printed words with and without auditory and gesture feedback.* Presented at the 3rd Annual Conference for Clinical Augmentative and Alternative Communication, Pittsburgh, PA.

Nelson, K. E. (1989). Strategies for first language teaching. In M. L. Rice & R. Schiefelbusch (Eds.), *The teachability of language* (pp. 263–310). Baltimore, MD: Paul H. Brookes.

Soto, G., & Toro-Zambrana, W. (1995). Investigation of Blissymbol use from a language research paradigm. *AAC: Augmentative and Alternative Communication, 11*(2), 118–130. Doi: 10.1080/07434619512331277219

Sutton, A. E., & Morford, J. P. (1998). Constituent order in picture pointing sequences produced by speaking children using AAC. *Applied Psycholinguistics, 19*(4), 525–536.

Todman, J., & Alm, N. (2003). Modeling conversational pragmatics in communication aids. *Journal of Pragmatics, 35*(4), 523–538.

Tomasello, M. (2003). *Constructing a language: A usage-based theory of language acquisition.* Cambridge, MA: Harvard University Press.

Valli, C., Lucas, C., & Mulrooney, K. J. (2005). *Linguistics of American Sign Language: An introduction* (4th ed.). Washington, DC: Clerc Books.

CHAPTER 8

AAC and Intervention with Acquired Communication Disorders

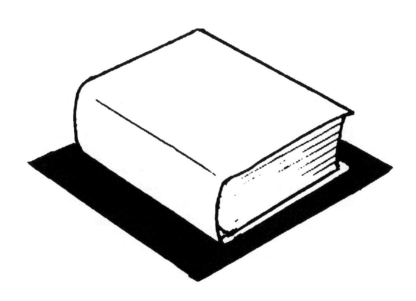

AN INCREASING PREVALENCE

In the past two decades, the number of individuals who use AAC has increased dramatically as the result of a number of factors: (1) improvement of general know-how about AAC among professionals, (2) advances in assistive technology, (3) more availability and accessibility of AAC, (4) decrease of resistance toward alternative forms of communication, and (5) a growing number of AAC candidates as a result of extended life expectancy and improvements of medical care services.

The last of these factors—AAC for individuals in later stages of the life span—is obviously obtaining an increasing importance. In the light of the emphasis on providing quality of life at every stage in life, communication is now generally considered to be a key factor for individuals in all stages of life and across all possible medical and psychological conditions. This chapter focuses on AAC solutions for individuals with acquired communication disorders, especially adults who have previously lived and functioned without disabilities but who experience sudden or progressive onset of communication limitations. Communication disorders are or can be a part of a whole range of acquired disorders, including aphasia, amyotrophic lateral sclerosis (ALS), Parkinson's disease, multiple sclerosis, Alzheimer's disease (AD) and other forms of dementia, traumatic brain injury (TBI), spinal cord injury, head and neck cancer, and brainstem impairment (including locked-in syndrome; Beukelman, Fager, Ball, & Dietz, 2007).

For the majority of adults with acquired communication disorders, the concern is somewhat different than for children who need AAC. Children's needs for augmentative communication are most often viewed in a developmental perspective. AAC solutions are defined differently according to whether children function at the level of a presymbolic communicator, a beginning communicator, a limited lexicon communicator, or a language-based communicator (Schlosser, 2003).

Garrett and Lasker (2013) have suggested classifications of AAC needs for individuals with severe aphasia that are based on different levels of partner-dependency and abilities to use aids (see section on aphasia later in this chapter). What most typologies of adult AAC users have in common are: (1) a focus on *communication* (i.e., whether we get the message across, rather than the form—linguistic or not), (2) a focus on *strategy* (resulting from an awareness that the communicators will have to do things "differently" as it is clear that the typical communication ways will insufficiently work), and (3) a focus on the *type of assistance* (the communication partner will play an important role, besides the aids that will be used).

In other words, AAC for adults will, in most cases, be a matter of finding ways to improve functional interaction with partners and the social environment. It

will be about striving for independence. Of course, AAC does have multiple applications that make it a great tool (or set of tools) not only to improve daily communication and functional use, but also for language therapy, for example, for individuals with acquired aphasia (see more about this later in this chapter). But for most of the later acquired communication disorders, the primary goal of intervention will be the highest possible level of independency through communication.

THE NATURE OF THE CONDITION: COGNITIVE, LINGUISTIC, OR MOTOR

The production of natural speech results from the coordinated use of cognitive, linguistic, and motor skills: a message originates in cognitive conception and planning (*cognition*), is shaped by grammar and lexical choices (*linguistics*), and is executed by a *motor* plan (in speech articulation).

What Is the *Linguistic* Nature of Disorder?

Aphasia is, by definition, a condition that affects the internal linguistic system. Depending on type and severity of the aphasia, a person will display some combination of expressive and receptive language problems, often with severe word finding difficulties, apraxia of speech, and/or syntactic problems. Individuals may also exhibit echolalia (the tendency to repeat words or phrases that one hears), word perseveration (the involuntary repetition of the same word after it has been produced once), and logorrhea (an uncontrollable flow of words). One needs to take this into account when trying to find AAC solutions for people with severe linguistic problems. A communication device that requires the person to construct linguistic messages (word by word selection) may not be appropriate. On the other hand, a condition such as ALS will primarily affect speech (and other motor executive functions) but not the internal language coding ability. AAC solutions for this condition will therefore include speech-generating devices.

What Is the Motor Nature of the Disorder?

Does the condition limit the range of motor actions a person can perform? Does this limit voluntary complex actions and motor planning (as in apraxia)? What are the alternative access modes (pointing, touching, eye gaze, and so on) that remain possible and can be brought under the person's control?

What Are the Cognitive Elements Affecting the Disorder?

Loss of memory is one of the characteristics that can be encountered in multiple conditions. We specifically need to pay attention to the possibility of word memory limitations. Word finding problems may possibly be of a different nature than generally decreased memory potential. Word finding is a limitation of the internal mental search function. Remember that, in typical speech, word identification (lexical access) needs to occur very fast. Individuals with word finding problems often indicate that they "know" the word but that they struggle with the so-called tip of the tongue phenomenon. AAC techniques can be valuable help for therapeutic training of individuals with severe word finding problems. By associating the word with other modalities (gestures, manual signs, a graphic symbol, or device-generated speech), the person can be taught techniques to self-activate the neuromotor patterns required for articulation of the word. No doubt, the most important cognitive aspects are the level of consciousness and awareness, and the ability to plan one's own actions.

Other Questions

Besides the characterization of the primary nature of the acquired disorder (cognitive, linguistic, or motor), two other important questions need to the addressed: the emotional/social factors and the progressive nature of the condition.

What Are the Emotional/Social Factors Involved—Both With the Client and His or Her Partners?

Motivation, social support, and the willingness to try and change a person's condition are strong determiners of success of intervention. Communication forms always have an influence on both the person who utters the message and the person who receives it. If a new way of expressing a message is introduced, partners will need to learn new "receptor strategies." In the first place, the communication partners will need to adjust their expectations. If they have become used to the fact that the person doesn't speak, they may have unconsciously developed the habit of not asking the person, or not waiting for a contribution in the conversation. Changing habits is not always easy, especially if specific ways of doing things have been established for a long time.

What Are the Progressive Characteristics Involved?

Yorkston and Beukelman (2007) emphasize that one cannot underestimate the impact of a progressive disorder such as Huntington's disease, multiple sclerosis, and Parkinson's disease. The progressive nature requires the persons and their communication partners to strike a balance between using the possibilities to communicate that are still available and the need to anticipate for a time when less muscular power and less muscular coordination will be possible.

Natural Speech

Depending on the nature of the impairment, natural speech will be affected in different ways. For example, *aphasia*, being a linguistic disorder, may be manifested by word finding problems, syntactic problems, and (linguistic) comprehension problems. *Dementias* can also be characterized by comprehension problems, but these will less likely be limited to retention and retrieval of solely linguistic information. *Acquired motor disorders* typically do not imply the existence of conceptual or comprehension problems. They essentially show limitations in executing a motor plan typically due to loss of neuromotor control (Figure 8–1).

When deciding on the best intervention and solution, it is important to keep in mind that functionality is what is needed: AAC should improve the quality of life, or open perspectives for rehabilitation. A functional approach implies that there is no such thing as "AAC for aphasia" which would be distinct from "AAC for TBI," or other conditions. When applying AAC, the practitioner will always need to propose solutions that are based on the assessment of condition and progress/evolution that is unique for each individual.

ACQUIRED COGNITIVE CHALLENGES

Dementia is a generic umbrella term that encompasses a variety of causes and configurations of symptoms. Contrary to ALS, the central challenge of dementia is the diminution of the cognitive executive function. Individuals who suffer from dementia will have most difficulties with the "cognitive" side of the message generating and interpreting process, that is, knowing what to say, finding the words, and interpreting the information they receive in relation to knowledge they have about their communication partner and about reality.

The most common and best-known form of dementia is Alzheimer's disease (AD) (Brill, 2005), often called the "forgetting disease" or "a disease that destroys parts of the brain." AD is usually characterized by a gradual deterioration of memory, awareness, and cognitive functions, typically starting when people are in their sixties. A second type of dementia is vascular dementia, which results from cerebrovascular infarcts, which can cause sudden changes in memory and cognitive behavior. Other forms include mixed dementia, fronto-temporal dementia, and dementia that can occur as part of Huntington's disease and Parkinson's disease (Holmes, 2012).

Although language and communication may not appear to be the central problem of dementia, some of the AAC techniques have shown to be extremely helpful (Bourgeois, Dijkstra, Burgio, & Allen-

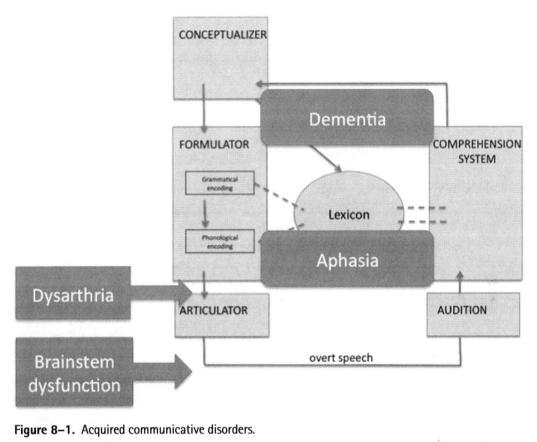

Figure 8–1. Acquired communicative disorders.

Burge, 2001; Bourgeois, Fried-Oken, & Rowland, 2010; Bourgeois & Hickey, 2007).

Tools that may be used to train or keep memory active include low-tech memory wallets/books, visualized schedules, and increasingly electronic organizers. People with dementia can benefit from the fact that many AAC materials are visible and tangible. Graphic symbols, organized in a schedule can be used as a reminder of the sequence of activities planned for the day. Graphic symbols can also be used to trigger access to internalized information. Additionally, basic speech-generating devices can add an auditory constituent. For example, one can use the speech-generating barcode reader (e.g., B.A.Bar,

Figure 8–2) to read prespoken messages on barcodes for self-reminders (e.g., an auditory "to-do" list).

Speech-generating devices can offer a combination of visual and auditory reminders. Speech output devices can be used as a spoken step-by-step guidance if a person needs to remember a sequence of activities. Together with a group of students at the University of Virginia, Braddock (McDaniel, Franzel, Koch, Peteron, & Braddock, 2009) conducted a study exploring training results of the use of a *sensory resource guide.* A sensory resource guide is a structured set of objects and pictures that serve as external memory aids. They carefully analyzed the training

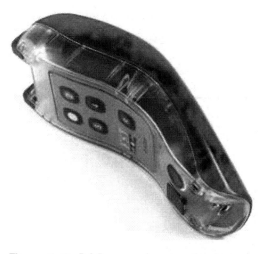

Figure 8–2. B.A.Bar speech generating barcode reader. Reproduced with permission.

results of three individuals who had been diagnosed with dementia. They concluded that these augmentatives do indeed offer possibilities to improve communication of the participants.

In all these cases, intervention is essentially an attempt to facilitate access to words, messages and other internal representations through a systematic linking with an alternative modality. Objects and graphic symbols are prime components for these AAC strategies. The latest mobile computing, tablet, and cell phone technology is offering a range of possibilities like automatic alarms, spoken reminders, screen visualization, one-key speed dial, and more.

ACQUIRED LINGUISTIC CHALLENGES

Aphasiology is the discipline that attempts to describe and categorize conditions that result from acquired brain lesions in brain areas that serve linguistic functions. There

are several types of aphasia. They all have in common that the sufferer experiences difficulties in the microgenesis and/or interpretation of linguistic utterances. Aphasia is an impairment of linguistic functions, although it often can cooccur with cognitive, motor, and/or perceptual difficulties.

For decades, different forms of AAC have been introduced for persons with *acquired aphasia* (King, Alarcon, & Rogers, 2007). Aphasia is, by definition, a linguistic disorder. Therefore, AAC solutions need to find a way to strengthen, use, or rehabilitate the remaining linguistic abilities in the person. In other words, AAC can be considered as a tool for therapy (see further in the chapter) or as a tool that circumvents linguistic communication.

Even though there are different types of aphasia and intervention that differ from client to client, generally, AAC intervention will focus on the following four intervention areas: (1) learning and training of new communication strategies by the client, (2) learning and training of new communication strategies by the client's communication partners (including relatives or coresidents), (3) improvement of word finding, and (4) help with message construction and narratives.

In planning the specifics of an intervention, Lasker, Garrett, and Fox (2007, p. 163) suggest that the following aspects should be taken into consideration:

- Determine type of communicator
- Conduct a needs assessment
- Conduct a modality assessment
- Conduct a role play
- Topic and vocabulary inventory
- Autobiographical information.

The authors indicate that it is important to see the differences between individuals who suffer from aphasia in a primarily *functional* way (i.e., by asking what they can accomplish through communication, how they do it (strategies), and how this can be improved. By assessing the functionality of those with aphasia, the authors propose the following typology:

■ *Basic-choice communicators* are individuals that may have a profound cognitive-linguistic disorder across modalities, but who may be able to respond to well-structured communicative messages—such as a choice between two options ("do you want tea or coffee?" while holding a bag of coffee in your right hand and a teabag in your other hand). Pointing to things or people in the environment and bringing the choices close to the person are all ways of

referencing to nonlinguistic elements, bringing the essential elements of the message to the perceivable foreground.

■ *Controlled-situation communicators* are individuals who may be able to function well if you structure the information through repetition and visualization. Often pen and paper (to write down words—much like a good school teacher would do on a blackboard to keep the student focused on specific concepts) will do a tremendous job. The communication partner may also bring in maps, pictures, and objects—to increase the concreteness of the interaction (Figure 8–3).

All the efforts to refer to external references can be opportunities to increase the chances that

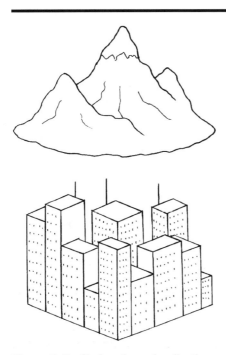
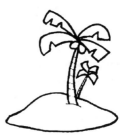

Figure 8–3. Choices from visualization.

the client will be able to access linguistic information. Indeed, word finding (access to the internal mental lexicon) can be triggered by stimuli in different modalities (pointing, objects, visual schemas, maps, pictures, written words):

■ *Comprehensive communicators* are generally able to activate speech and language but often fail when it comes to exerting linguistic control to self-monitor their own speech. Comprehensive communicators may get lost in word repetitions, or may produce involuntarily irrelevant or incoherent speech segments. These individuals need communication partners that can help them with linguistic monitoring: they may help by cueing words or phrases, by indicating a clear turn-taking alternation, and by visualizing parts of the content of the conversation.

■ *Augmented-input communicators* are individuals with aphasia who find it hard to process language that is directed to them directly, without support of additional information. For these individuals, the key is to be multimodal: use pictures, manual signs, repetition, words on display screens, or any other strategies that will bring the linguistic information to the foreground. Augmented-input communicators can use an instruction card that explains communication partners about their need to receive structured and multimodal information.

■ *Specific-need communicators* are those speakers who may have developed reasonable skills to get through the day, but who have difficulties in specific situations. They might need specific techniques such as yes-no questioning ("please ask me questions that I can answer with yes or no"), or, like augmented-input communicators, use specifically prepared communication cards.

ACQUIRED MOTOR IMPAIRMENT

A number of acquired impairments primarily affect the execution of motor functions. Complex fine motor patterns, such as speech articulation, often suffer in conditions where a person loses control over motor patterns.

Amyotrophic Lateral Sclerosis

The term Amyotrophic Lateral Sclerosis (ALS: sometimes called Lou Gehrig's disease; Mitsumoto, Przedborski, Gordon, & Ralph Erskine Conrad Memorial Fund, 2006) or *ALS* refers to the fact that there is a lack of nourishment of the muscles (*amyotrophy*) situated at the *lateral* part of the spinal cord that results in hardening (*sclerosis*) of the spinal cord. It is a condition that affects both the upper and the lower motor neurons, and that leads to degeneration and loss of motor control. Individuals with ALS gradually lose natural speech. As a pure motor disorder—not a language or cognitive disorder—the individual's potential to think, understand language, and internally use language remains preserved. Probably the best-known person with ALS, who uses AAC, is Stephen Hawking, the world-famous British theoretical physicist. Hawking has lived with ALS for decades, which makes him the most protracted case of ALS ever known. After onset of the disease, a person usually dies within next 10 years. Although it is certainly not his field of study, Hawking has probably done more to promote AAC worldwide to make it an acceptable form of communication.

Communication solutions for ALS clients (Ball, Beukelman, & Bardach, 2007) include voice amplification, conversation repair strategies, alphabet supplementation, and the use of speech-generating devices. In preparation of the stage in which the use of a speech-generating device will be a necessity, more and more ALS patients will resort to voice banking. Voice banking consists of recording a series of messages with the patient's voice before it becomes too weak or too slurred to be usable. The client will record messages such as "yes," "no," as well as those like, "how are you doing today?" and "glad to see you." It is also crucially important to have messages like, "My mouth is dry," "I have no appetite," I need my glasses," "Give me a tissue, please," "Clean my mouth," "Sorry, I am having difficulty breathing," "I need suctioning." Advances in computer electronic measuring and recording of human speech acoustics are allowing us now to create digitized speech that includes all the characteristics of the person's original voice. This is based on detailed spectrographic analysis of speech samples of the person. The obtained speech characteristics are then entered as variables into the speech-generating device (Spiegel, 2013).

Brainstem Dysfunction

Brainstem dysfunction, locked-in syndrome, and the possible solutions for these conditions made available by AAC have received mainstream attention in the past decade, essentially because of the dramatic and frightening nature of the maladies. Damage to the central nervous system structures that are located in the brainstem typically affects the motor executive functions of speech to a profound extent. The impairment is the result of an acquired condition. In most of the cases, it is a *brainstem stroke*, involving a disruption of the blood supply provided to the brainstem by the basilar artery. Occlusion of the artery is the most common cause. Many individuals with brainstem impairment experience anarthria—an inability to speak. Most people with brainstem dysfunction will require some form of AAC, at least initially.

The most dramatic condition is, without any doubt, the locked-in syndrome (LIS) or *ventral pontine syndrome*. This is a severe motor impairment in which an individual is conscious but quadriplegic. Voluntary movement is limited to eye movements or eye blinks. For some people with LIS, only vertical eye movements are available. LIS usually occurs as a result of brainstem stroke; however, it occasionally results from severe TBI. Some authors identify individuals as having incomplete LIS if the individuals have severe brainstem damage but are able to move their head or an upper extremity. The syndrome attracted worldwide attention after the 1997 publication of the (French) book "Le scaphandre et le papillon" (The Diving Bell and the Butterfly) by Jean-Dominique Bauby (Crumley, 1997). This publication was and still is remarkable for a number of reasons. Jean-Dominique Bauby used to be a leading member of the Parisian jet set. Before his stroke, he had been a trendy journalist and writer, editor of the French fashion magazine *ELLE*. The stroke left him incapable of any movement, with the exception of eye blinking with the right eye. Using the letter-by-letter partner assistive technique with his treating speech-language pathologist Sandrine Fichou, Bauby dictated his book, the amazing and touching story of his condition. The book demonstrates the enormous creative power and courage that individuals in a locked-in situation can generate. In 2007, the movie with the same title was produced.

In the movie adaptation, the French-Canadian actor Marie-Josée Croze plays speech-language pathologist Sandrine who introduces the idea to use an eye blinking code and a letter board. Despite the initial frustration, Bauby understands that this is his only and last chance to be a writer and send a message to the world. He does so by dictating the manuscript of the book, first to Sandrine and further to ghostwriter Claude Mendibil. The film, issued in 2007, is a mixture of facts and fiction, but still renders an impressive picture of the locked-in condition (Mathiasen, 2008). Bauby died just 10 days after the publication of the book. One of the great merits of his book and his courage, together with the people around him, is the fact that he brought attention to the locked-in condition, as well as the possibilities of AAC. In his book, he renders homage to the work of speech-language pathologists, whom he calls angels.

In the past decade and a half, many patients with locked-in syndrome have found tremendous help in the use of advanced eye-gaze systems (see Chapters 2 and 3). The developments of applications of Brain-Computer Interaction (BCI) hold even more promise for the future. BCI is an advanced form of access to a device (a computer) via pulses that are registered through a brain implant. Anything that can take individuals with locked-in syndrome out of their isolation will be an improvement in their quality of life.

Other Acquired Predominantly Motor Disorders

Several other conditions can be the cause of severe limitations or loss of the possibility of natural speech articulation. These include (but are not limited to) *spinal cord injury* and *Traumatic Brain Injury (TBI)*.

Spinal Cord Injury

The spinal cord is "the gateway for information transfer between body and brain, as well as a center for neuronal circuits that integrate and coordinate complex sensory, motor, and autonomic functions" (Hochman, 2007). Generally speaking, body movements and sensations of the areas that are connected with the spinal cord below where the injury has occurred become severely limited or impossible. Depending on the level of damage, natural speech can be difficult, essentially because the person has no longer the possibility to regulate subglottal air pressure, which is needed for natural speech. AAC can be a solution, including the use of partner-dependent strategies (e.g., yes-no questions) and devices/computers to which the person has accessibility (e.g., voice recognition, dictation software or a form of Brain-Computer Interaction, see Ikegami, Takano, Saeki, and Kansaku [2011]).

Traumatic Brain Injury

TBI is "an alteration in brain function, or other evidence of brain pathology, caused by an external force" (Brain Injury Association of America, 2012). TBI can be the result of physical violence, traffic, or other accidents (Abelson-Mitchell, 2013), and can occur at all ages, but the highest prevalence is in the late adolescence and during early adulthood years. Recovery depends on multiple factors (degree and location of injury, nature of intervention, cognitive and linguistic levels of functioning). A permanent disability, including the possibility of speech and communication limitations, is often to be reckoned with. Depending on the person's level of functioning, AAC can provide an important help in regaining, improving, or establishing quality of life (Fager, Doyle, & Karantounis, 2007).

Head and Neck Cancer

Head and neck cancer is a term used to indicate cancers of the upper aerodigestive tract. They can be cancers in the nasal cavity, the pharynx, the oral cavity, and the larynx. These are critical areas for the production of natural speech. Cancer intervention may include surgical removal of parts of the anatomical structures (e.g., glossectomy or layngectomy), which will severely impact natural speech production. Alternative ways of speaking and communicating are (a combination of) esophageal speech (Diedrich, Youngstrom, & Youngstrom, 1966), the use of an electrolarynx (Herrmann & Amatsu,

1986), and the use of speech-generating devices (Rodriguez & Blischak, 2010; Rodriguez & Rowe, 2010; Sullivan, Gaebler, & Ball, 2007).

AAC AS THERAPY AND REHABILITATION TOOL

AAC tools can be used to establish and improve daily communication needs of individuals with acquired conditions. They can also be employed in therapeutic intervention to improve communication and linguistic skills. As we have discussed, AAC is used regularly as a form of *direct communication*, but it is also used as a *therapy tool* for those with aphasia. One therapy objective for which AAC can be helpful is word finding. *Word finding problems* are often at the core of the aphasia problem. The internal mental routes to the mental lexicon are obstructed, or the person with aphasia has trouble on the way "from the mind to the mouth."

The use of nonspeech modalities can sometimes be helpful in activating access to the lexicon. By associating the word with other modalities (gestures, manual signs, device-generated speech), the person can be taught techniques to self-activate the neuromotor patterns required for articulation of the word. Loncke, Kaulback, Meyer, Huber, and Nobis-Bosch (2006) compared the treatment effects of presenting individuals with aphasia with picture cards that contained: (1) the first phoneme of the word that could be activated by a barcode reader (this would serve as the first cue; Figure 8–4), (2) the whole word spoken that could be activated by the use of a barcode reader (this would serve as the second cue), and (3) no

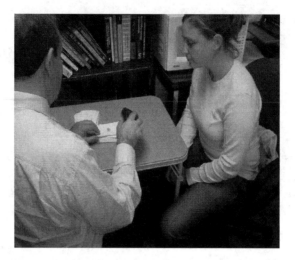

Figure 8–4. Speech stimulus material with speech-generating barcode reader.

additional speech information (traditional cues were used here).

The study was run with three participants, all of whom showed a severe acquired aphasia with word finding problems. The results showed that the participant(s) trained with words with the use of a barcode reader showed significantly better improvement than those trained with traditional cues.

In all these cases, intervention is essentially an attempt to facilitate access to words, messages, and other internal representations through a systematic linking with an alternative modality. Objects and graphic symbols are prime components for these AAC strategies. Additionally, basic speech-generating devices can add an auditory constituent. For example,

one can use the speech-generating barcode reader B.A.Bar to read prespoken messages on barcodes for self-reminders (e.g., an auditory "to-do" list).

SHORT-TERM AND LONG-TERM GOALS

Upon planning the intervention, one must set appropriate long-term and short-term goals. Both types of goals are (or should be) dictated by the need to raise or maintain a person's quality of life. Things to consider in planning the intervention include:

1. The role of the partners. Often, the spouse or life partner of the client

will almost have to be involved in the therapy as much as the client.

2. The interaction techniques and learning strategies used to change the patterns of learning and interaction. Typical strategies are, the use of *visualization* (making things visual, sometimes by using a drawing interactive pen-and-paper conversation), the use of *questions* as prompts, and the use of *choices* (a way of reducing the person's need to structure his/her answer—a kind of conversational multiple choice).

Effects of (Partially) Device–Based Language Therapy

There is a long tradition of low-tech intervention (often paper-and-pencil) in aphasia therapy. In the past 10 years, high-tech devices are increasingly used because of their better portability, lowering costs, and possibilities of self-training. The use of computer-devices is an excellent platform to create a wide range of therapeutic lesson plans and exercises. An excellent model is the Lingraphica™, a computer with programs especially designed to meet the communication and language needs of people suffering from aphasia. The exercises of the Lingraphica are not limited to the realm of word or short-message production, but also include sentence construction. The packet contains further a multimodal representation part that links pictures, words, and video clips together.

Devices can play a role in making sure that clients will effectively use the skills that have been acquired in therapy in daily life. We have certainly not yet exhausted all the possibilities of devices for individuals with aphasia. We should think more about how we can improve the functionality of our interventions hence the quality of life of our clients (Steele, Aftonomos, & Koul, 2010).

My former colleague Barbara Braddock and her associates (e.g., Rosenthal, Braddock, Loncke, & Turner, 2009) set up a study to explore if a person with acquired aphasia would be able to use a speech-generating device as a means of self-directed speech to structure her thinking and planning. They conducted a single subject design study with a 61-year-old female participant, who was diagnosed with nonfluent Broca aphasia. At the time of the intervention, the participant was 5 years post onset. At the time of pretesting, the home environment was modified by barcodes that had been placed on selected objects that were part of the person's daily routines. Forty barcodes were placed based on the participant's preference and the designated phrases were recorded. For example, a barcode was attached to the coffee maker. The participant was then instructed how to operate the barcode reader and asked to use it repetitively on a daily basis. During 4 weeks, a 1-hour home intervention session was conducted. This consisted of reviewing the barcodes in her home and encouraging her to use the AAC in multiple contexts (i.e., over the phone, logbook cues, etc.). The improvements in this participant led the researchers to conclude that, indeed: (1) AAC devices that offer an auditory feedback may have an effect on internal phonological reinforcement for practiced items, and (2)—specifically—that bound morphological markers, the little word endings for example, appear the most sensitive to change in speech production.

Interactive technology continues to hold enormous promise for intervention and self-therapy for individuals with acquired disorders. This has been demonstrated for people with acquired aphasia, especially persons with preserved cognitive functions (Aftonomos, Steele, & Wertz, 1997).

Acceptability

A crucial aspect of introducing AAC for individuals with aphasia or other acquired communication disorders is the acceptability of AAC and the alternative forms of communication. Accepting AAC, learning to use the new ways of communication, and integrating it into a person's daily life, is often associated with an acceptance of the functional status/condition in which the person sees himself/herself presently and in the future. This may be psychologically a hard step to take, for it is something related to the self-image of the person and to expectations met and unmet, and to dreams fulfilled or unfulfilled. Just like a wheelchair may become a symbol of stagnation in the eyes of the individual who has lost mobility, the communication device may be the symbol of the fact that the person will "have to settle for less." This can be confrontational, not only for the persons themselves, but also for their communication partners and loved ones.

TELEPRACTICE, SELF-THERAPY, AND DISTANCE INTERVENTION

A speech-generating device may also have the advantage of allowing self-training. Nobis-Bosch and her colleagues (2006) asked a 55-year-old adult male with aphasia to enter a self-training program in which he would practice independently on a daily basis. They found that the use of the speech-generating barcode reader was more efficient than the traditional paper-and-pencil tasks. Practice via direct auditory stimulation as provided by a speech-generating barcode reader was more favorable than indirect stimulation via written input (word reading). For both methods, the frequency of stimulation was extremely high. Apparently, frequency of stimulation irrespective of the stimulation method made specific items more available to the mental lexicon.

These studies have supported that the use of speech-generating devices for self-training has the following advantages: (1) consistent feedback (you hear exactly the same word/message each time you activate the device), (2) relative easiness to handle (depending on the device, it can be programmed that it just requires the use of one single button—or, in the case of the barcode reader, holding the device over the barcode and letting it scan and speak), and (3) frequent self-exposure (one can repeat and practice the same word/messages over and over again).

CONCLUSION

It is to be expected that the need for AAC by individuals with acquired speech (or other) disorders will continue to increase in the next decades. AAC solutions can be an important contribution to restoration or improvement of quality of life.

POINTS TO REMEMBER

■ The prevalence of acquired disorders that imply AAC needs has increased over the past decades. This growth will probably continue.

- The nature of an acquired disorder can be motor, linguistic, cognitive, or a combination of these.
- When determining the AAC needs of a person with acquired disorders, social and emotional factors need to be considered.
- Intervention decisions need to be based on consideration of quality of life.
- Intervention decisions need to take into consideration the projected development (including the possible progressive nature) of the disorder and the needs.
- AAC needs for individuals with acquired aphasia can be described according to the following typology: basic-choice communicators, controlled-situation communicators, comprehensive communicators, augmented-input communicators, and specific needs communicators.
- Eye-gaze access systems have been a tremendous help for clients with locked-in syndrome.
- AAC tools can be employed to aid in reaching language therapy goals (e.g., word finding facilitation).
- AAC tools can be used in self-therapy, telepractice, and distance therapy.

REFERENCES

Abelson-Mitchell, N. (2013). *Neurotrauma*. Chicester, UK: Wiley.

Aftonomos, L. B., Steele, R. D., & Wertz, R. T. (1997). Promoting recovery in chronic aphasia with an interactive technology. *Archives of Physical Medicine and Rehabilitation, 78*(8), 841–846.

Ball, L., Beukelman, D., & Bardach, L. (2007). Amyotrophic lateral sclerosis. In D. Beukelman, K. Garrett, & K. Yorkston (Eds.), *Augmentative communication strategies for adults with acute and chronic medical Conditions* (pp. 287–345). Baltimore, MD: Paul H. Brookes.

Beukelman, D. R., Fager, S., Ball, L., & Dietz, A. (2007). AAC for adults with acquired neurological conditions: A review. *Augmentative and Alternative Communication, 23*(3), 230–242.

Bourgeois, M., Dijkstra, K., Burgio, L., & Allen-Burge, R. (2001). Memory aids as an augmentative and alternative communication strategy for nursing home residents with dementia. *Augmentative and Alternative Communication, 17*(3), 196–210.

Bourgeois, M., Fried-Oken, M., & Rowland, C. (2010). AAC strategies and tools for persons with dementia. *ASHA Leader, 15*(3), 8–11.

Bourgeois, M., & Hickey, E. (2007). Dementia. In D. Beukelman, K. Garrett, & K. Yorkston (Eds.), *Augmentative communication strategies for adults with acute or chronic medical conditions* (pp. 243–285). Baltimore, MD: Paul H. Brookes.

Brain Injury Association of America. (2012). *BIAA adopts new TBI definition*. Retrieved from http://www.biausa.org/announcements/biaa-adopts-new-tbi-definition

Brill, M. T. (2005). *Alzheimer's disease*. New York, NY: Benchmark Books.

Crumley, B. (1997). A triumph of the spirit. *Time, 149*(12), 90.

Diedrich, W. M., Youngstrom, K. A., & Youngstrom, K. A. (1966). *Alaryngeal speech*. Springfield, IL: Thomas.

Fager, S., Doyle, M., & Karantounis, R. (2007). Traumatic brain injury. In D. Beukelman, K. Garrett, & K. Yorkston (Eds.), *Augmentative communication strategies for adults with acute or chronic medical conditions* (pp. 131–162). Baltimore, MD: Paul H. Brookes.

Garrett, K., & Lasker, J. (2013). Adults with severe aphasia and apraxia of speech. In D. Beukelman & P. Mirenda (Eds.), *Augmentative and alternative communication supporting children and adults with complex communication needs* (4th ed., pp. 405–445). Baltimore, MD: Paul H. Brookes.

Herrmann, I. F., & Amatsu, M. (1986). *Speech restoration via voice prostheses*. Berlin, Germany: Springer-Verlag.

Hochman, S. (2007). Spinal cord. *Current Biology,* *17*(22), R950–R955.

Holmes, C. (2012). Dementia. *Medicine; Psychiatry: Part 1 of 2, 40*(11), 628–631.

Ikegami, S., Takano, K., Saeki, N., & Kansaku, K. (2011). Operation of a P300-based brain–computer interface by individuals with cervical spinal cord injury. *Clinical Neurophysiology, 122*(5), 991–996.

King, J., Alarcon, N., & Rogers, M. (2007). Primary progressive aphasia. In D. Beukelman, K. Garrett, & K. Yorkston (Eds.), *Augmentative communication strategies for adults with acute or chronic medical conditions* (pp. 207–241). Baltimore, MD: Paul H. Brookes.

Lasker, J., Garrett, K., & Fox, L. (2007). Severe aphasia. In D. Beukelman, K. Garrett, & K. Yorkston (Eds.), *Augmentative communication strategies for adults with acute or chronic medical conditions* (pp. 163–206). Baltimore, MD: Paul H. Brookes.

Loncke, F., Kaulback, L., Meyer, L., Huber, W., & Nobis-Bosch, R. (2006). *How effective can speech-generating devices be in aphasia therapy?* Paper presented at the Biennial Conference of the International Society for Augmentative and Alternative Communication, Dusseldorf, Germany.

Mathiasen, H. (2008). Mind over body: The diving bell and the butterfly. *The American Journal of Medicine, 121*(9), 829.

McDaniel, J., Franzel, M., Koch, H., Peteron, J., & Braddock, B. (2009). *The use of a sensory resource guide in dementia care.* Paper presented at the 3rd Annual Conference for Clinical Augmentative and Alternative Communication, Pittsburgh, PA.

Mitsumoto, H., Przedborski, S., Gordon, P. H., & Ralph Erskine Conrad Memorial Fund. (2006). *Amyotrophic lateral sclerosis.* New York, NY: Taylor & Francis.

Nobis-Bosch, R., Radermacher, I., Springer, L., & Huber, W. (2006). *Supervised home training in Aphasia: Application of the electronic language trainer B.A.Bar—A single case study.* Paper presented at the International Aphasia Rehabilitation Conference, Sheffield, UK.

Rodriguez, C. S., & Blischak, D. M. (2010). Communication needs of nonspeaking hospitalized postoperative patients with head and neck cancer. *Applied Nursing Research, 23*(2), 110–115.

Rodriguez, C., & Rowe, M. (2010). Use of a speech-generating device for hospitalized postoperative patients with head and neck cancer experiencing speechlessness. *Oncology Nursing Forum, 37*(2), 199–205.

Rosenthal, R., Braddock, B., Loncke, F., & Turner, K. (2009). *Effectiveness of a speech-generating device: Patterns of use and restorative speech in adults with nonfluent aphasia.* Research presentation at the Speech-Language-Hearing Association of Virginia Annual Conference, Richmond, VA.

Schlosser, R. W. (2003). *The efficacy of augmentative and alternative communication: Toward evidence-based practice.* San Diego, CA: Academic Press.

Spiegel, A. (2013, March 11). *New voices for the voiceless: Synthetic speech gets an upgrade.* NPR Radio Report.

Steele, R., Aftonomos, L., & Koul, R. (2010). Outcome improvements in persons with chronic global aphasia following the use of a speech-generating device. *Acta Neuropsychologica, 8*(4), 342–359.

Sullivan, M., Gaebler, C., & Ball, L. (2007). AAC for people with head and neck cancer. In D. Beukelman, K. Garrett, & K. Yorkston (Eds.), *Augmentative communication strategies for adults with acute or chronic medical conditions* (pp. 347–367). Baltimore, MD: Paul H. Brookes.

Yorkston, K., & Beukelman, D. (2007). AAC intervention for progressive conditions. In D. Beukelman, K. Garrett, & K. Yorkston (Eds.), *Augmentative communication strategies for adults with acute or chronic medical conditions* (pp. 317–345). Baltimore, MD: Paul H. Brookes.

CHAPTER 9

AAC and Literacy Development

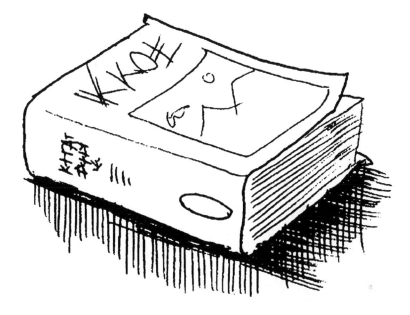

Why should we pay special attention to the development and the maintenance of literacy skills for individuals who need or use AAC? There are several reasons. First and most importantly, individuals who use AAC pose an interesting question concerning learning processes that are involved in learning to read and write. How does the fact that one does not speak influence the understanding of phonics (i.e., the systematic sound—letter connections on which alphabet writing is based)? Do you need to be able to "sound out" words to learn to read them? If that were the case, AAC users have an enormous problem. Fortunately, AAC users can and do acquire literacy, but educators need to approach it in a strategic way (Scherz & Hart, 2002). At any rate, the unique (or at least different) conditions in which AAC users find themselves when it comes to learning to read and write, invite a neurocognitive approach (Van Balkom & Verhoeven, 2010); which are the internal representations (are they multimodal?—see also Chapter 5—and how is reading processed? How does a reader compose meaning while reading?, Is this a parallel process of both semantic and phonological decoding?)

Second, the development of literacy skills only fairly recently became a focus in the intervention planning for AAC users. In the early years of AAC, all attention went to enabling direct face-to-face communicative interaction. Literacy development was not so much in the focus or may not always even have been considered to even be a possibility. Hence, our research and intervention programs need to "catch up" and provide effective literacy curricula for AAC users.

The third reason is that AAC users may use literacy skills as compensatory and supplemental strategies more often than non-AAC users. AAC users may, therefore, have an even greater vested interest in literacy. To put it in simple words: if you can speak less, you may want to compensate by writing more! In how far is this an attainable goal? Let's explore these ideas in this chapter.

LITERACY ACQUISITION AND AAC USE: AN INTERESTING RELATION

In typical development, children acquire language through speech in a natural, interactive way years before they will become skilled in literacy. Learning to read implies the ability to reflect on spoken words (a metalinguistic skill) and discover that they can be analyzed as sequences of sounds, which can be spatially represented as strings of letters. Learning this skill requires the systematic teaching of phonics. Natural speech comes first, after which children proceed to learning literacy-related skills once they have some metalinguistic skills. For example, children will understand that a word consists of parts (the sounds of the spoken word, the letters of the written word) and that a "longer" word consists of more letters, referring to more sounds (phonemes).

Interestingly, children who are provided with a communication board or an AAC device at a very young age will often encounter graphic symbols at a relatively early stage in language development. Two- or three-year old children can learn to point to a graphic symbol (often a picture) to indicate that they are hungry, that they want to play a game, or that they are tired and want to have a rest. Typically developing non-AAC users don't use writing to tell you something until they are 6 or 7 years old (or older). This difference between early graphic symbol users and typically developing children is interesting. Could it be that, by providing graphic symbol communication to young AAC users, we give them a developmental advantage when it comes to reading and writing? After all, reading and writing is precisely that: the use of graphic symbols (letters, printed words). Sadly enough, this does not seem to be the case; among AAC users, many do have a significant delay in acquiring literacy (Dahlgren Sandberg, Smith, & Larsson, 2010). In response to this finding, in the past 15 years, several educators and speech-language pathologists have decided to make the promotion of literacy for AAC users their main field of work.

To further analyze this problem, it is helpful to identify the skills that a graphic symbol user employs in communicating. For example, suppose you are trying to teach a child to indicate when he or she needs to use the bathroom by pointing to a picture of a toilet. To aid his or her learning, the clinician may place the printed sentence, "I need to use the bathroom," underneath the picture. In addition, a graphic symbol of a toilet is placed on a speech-generating device producing the spoken output. If the child is able to indicate his or her need to use the restroom through the facilitation of the given strategies, what does it tell us about his or her abilities? First, it is an indication that the child has understood the basic principle of communication—you do something (i.e., point to a symbolic picture) in order to obtain something. It may be the result of some associative learning, which does not necessarily imply that the child grasps the pictorial meaning (the iconicity may or may not be a factor that facilitates the learning process). It may be simply that the child has learned that this specific location on the board leads to the right result. In this situation, to make sure that the child pays attention to the picture, one can experiment with placing a different picture in the same location. If you put the picture of a hamburger in the "bathroom" location on the board, will the child still use that for bathroom requests? If so, it would be an indication of one of the following: (1) the child may not yet be able to decode the picture as such; or (2) the child had already learned the location of the picture as a motor response and did not expect you to move it to test him or her and to disrupt a previously learned motor plan.

A HELP OR A BARRIER?

Is the use of graphic symbols a blessing on the way to literacy or does it hinder progress to full literacy? Does your understanding of graphic symbols help you comprehend what it means to "read," to break down written sentences and words into parts? Or does it leave you at some kind of general graphic-pictorial level without feeling pushed to discover a more abstract orthographic principle? (i.e., written words consist of letters that have some systematic relation with the phonemes/sounds you can perceive). McNaughton

and Lindsay (1995) were among the first who formulated this intriguing issue and suggested that "one should remain open to the possibility of a differential impact upon beginning reading due to use of different types of graphic representational systems" (p. 212).

THREE ABILITIES AND LEVELS OF GRAPHIC SYMBOL USE

As we question if graphic symbols can be used as a stepping-stone toward more literacy use, let us first look at the three levels of graphic symbol use.

1. The Ability to Pay Attention to Specifics of a Pictorial Representation

When do typically developing children start paying attention to pictures and their details? Is a bottle with a label containing a picture of a child in any way different than a bottle without that label? Babies live in an environment where many objects are pictorial, but there is little evidence that they notice any specific characteristics of these objects until they are in their second year of life. Interestingly, young children appear to have the capacity at a very young age—even as infants (and to a certain degree as newborns)—to discriminate between pictures of objects and the actual objects. Infants also have the capacity to recognize familiar objects and persons in photographs (DeLoache, Pierroutsakos, & Troseth, 1996). However amazing these early recognition skills may be, they are not sufficient for the complex use that is required in picture communication.

2. The Ability to Understand the Referential–Pictorial Meaning of a Graphic Symbol

DeLoache and colleagues (DeLoache, Pierroutsakos, & Uttal, 2003) talk about "pictorial competence," which refers to "the many factors involved in perceiving, interpreting, understanding, and using pictures" (p. 114). Their research shows that "understanding a picture" for a young child is far from easy or evident. They argue that mental representation, underlying the use of a symbol, is always a dual representation: one of the referent and one of the symbol itself. Children go through different stages before arriving at the "adult" way of understanding pictures. For example, 18-month-olds appear not to be bothered at all if they are presented with pictures in an upside-down orientation. Interestingly, this is not because they do not have a sense to interpret orientation. They tend to "correct" objects that are presented in an inverted position. It takes a maturation—and probably enculturation—process before children spontaneously turn the picture into the right position.

3. The Ability to Insert a Pictorial Representation in a Meaningful Way in a Sequence of Actions

Within AAC, the use of picture-exchange is probably the best-known practice to turn a graphic symbol into something that is part of a real communicative act. The graphic symbol is used as a communicative symbol that gets you something accomplished through interaction. The first stage in the Picture Exchange Communication system (PECS) is "How to Communicate" (Bondy & Frost, 1994), where the child is trained to pick up a picture and physically release it in the communicative partner's open hand. It is a learning process that essentially aims at making the communicative act a tangible event—where the message is not an abstract, invisible concept, but a physical object. The authors emphasize that this initial training is not necessarily a real communicative act from the perspective of the learner: It is meant to provide the learner with a behavior pattern that can be turned into a genuine communicative interaction. After Stage 1, the following stages in the PECS approach are (Phase 2) Distance and Persistence (overcoming barriers), (Phase 3) Discrimination Between Symbols (consequences between choices), (Phase 4) Using Phrases (I want . . . I see), (Phase 5) Answering a Direct Question (What do you see?), and (Phase 6) Commenting. One of the merits of this system is that the developers have provided us with a description that makes it clear that communicating with pictures involves an integration of intentionality, pragmatic skills, and physical skills.

CAN GRAPHIC SYMBOLS AID WORD RECOGNITION THROUGH ASSOCIATION?

Besides the question of whether the use of graphic symbols may induce some general underlying graphic and print awareness that can become useful for literacy development, one can wonder if there is another associative way to connect graphic understanding with learning to recognize and decode printed words.

Here we are referring to the common practice to print the word underneath or above the picture (Figure 9–1).

Does the child learn the written word "baby" when using the graphic symbol? Does it help to promote literacy if the sentence, "I need to go to the bathroom" is printed underneath the picture? One might argue that, after all, each time the child looks at this graphic symbol, he or she "sees" the message. Could it be that there is some passive learning that will help the child gradually access and understand the way print works? Would it be sufficient to have the printed words under the graphic symbol for the user to "recognize" the printed word and somehow pick up on the principles of orthography? There is not much evidence that supports such a hypothesis (although, to my knowledge, it has never been tested directly). Do typically developing children spontaneously notice the characteristics of written language in similar conditions? It appears that the answer is no: Justice, Skibbe, Canning, and Lankford (2005) tracked the eye gaze of preschool children looking at picture-salient versus print-salient books. They found that children spent more eye-gazing time with print when the books were more print-salient. This may already suggest one interpretation of our practices in AAC: if we want to take advantage of the fact that graphic symbols can be part of a multimodal configuration (the multimodal configuration would consist here of: the graphic symbol (pictorial representation), the printed word (orthographic representation), and speech output (auditory representation), we will need to draw the user's attention to it. Otherwise, the printed word may just be visual noise that is simply ignored by the learner.

ARE THE GRAPHIC SYMBOLS A HELP TO LITERACY?

Is there a conclusion we can draw from research: (1) whether the use of graphic symbols is or is not a help for literacy development, and (2) what should be done to transition from graphic symbols to a more traditional orthographic learning approach? Unfortunately, we are not aware of any research that explicitly investigates this question. It would be worthwhile though, and it could be the entry point for a productive educational practice for AAC users who have had experience with graphic symbols.

Maybe we should further operationalize this question. Specifically, one could ask whether specific graphic symbol systems would lend themselves more to literacy preparation than others. Note that

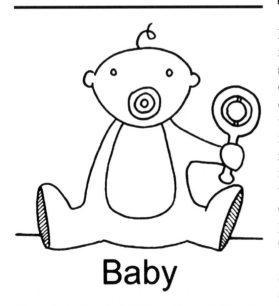

Baby

Figure 9–1. A typical AAC graphic symbol has the name of the symbol printed on it.

we here use the term symbol *systems* (as opposed to *sets*). In earlier chapters, we have described a system of graphic symbols as a collection of symbols that contain internal organizing principles—sets of rules on which users can rely to generate and recognize the symbols. Traditional orthography is perhaps the most salient case of a graphic symbol system—where the symbols (the written words) are entirely defined by the orthographic (spelling) rules. Blissymbolics or Blisswords (see Chapter 4) is an AAC system that uses a limited set of basic shapes that are combined and recombined to form graphic symbols. The user can rely on rule awareness to store and retrieve symbols. In other words, Blissymbolics contains a "sublexical" level (a level smaller than the entire symbol), somewhat similar to the sublexical "grapheme" level of written words. Does this entice the user to employ different strategies than if a *set* of graphic symbols would be used? We have no information whether the specific characteristics of Blissymbolics do have an influence on literacy development, but it would be interesting to find out.

Along similar lines, one could look whether the use of Minspeak (or Unity) would be beneficial for the acquisition of reading and writing. Minspeak (see Chapter 2) is a system that allows the user to generate words and messages through *icon sequencing*. The essence of icon sequencing is that the user accesses the symbol through a code (that has been learned through practice and that is often reflected in a motor pattern—much like typical users have learned typing keyboard motor patterns). Here again, one could ask the (research) question whether using a code (and a rule) would be beneficial for achieving literacy. These are fascinating research questions, with a major implication for the development of literacy intervention programs.

LITERACY ACTIVITIES AND A LITERACY CURRICULUM FOR AAC USERS

In typically developing children, one can describe the progression in reading skills and literacy as a continuous process going through different stages. For typically developing students, the following sequence has been suggested by reading education specialists and researchers such as Chall (1983):

Prereading Stage: Unsystematic accumulation of understandings about reading between preschool and kindergarten.

Stage 1: Initial Reading or Decoding Stage (Grades 1–2; Ages 6–7)

Stage 2: Confirmation, Fluency, Ungluing from Print, Automaticity Stage (Grades 2–3; Ages 7–8)

Stage 3: Reading for Learning (Grades 4–8; Ages 9–13)

Stage 4: Multiple Viewpoints Stage: (High School; Ages 14–18)

Stage 5: Construction and Reconstruction Stage (College; Ages 18 & up)

Understanding the stages and the processes involved is important as it affects curricular planning and decisions for children who use AAC. These decisions involve adaptations in how the regular curriculum is implemented, including compensating for the student's lack of access to oral production (Light & McNaughton, 2009). Erickson and Clendon (2009) are among a group of scholars who make a convincing case for a careful and strong literacy curriculum for young AAC users: "For students with AAC needs, the role of literacy extends beyond traditional access to content and demonstrating understanding in general. Although (graphic) symbols can meet a wide range of communication needs, the alphabet is the only symbol set that allows an individual to communicate precisely across environments and partners" (p. 195).

DIFFERENT CHALLENGES AT DIFFERENT STAGES

One can easily see why the practices for children who are AAC users can be challenging.

At the *pre-reading stage*, typically developing children learn and experience a multitude of activities and games that refer to graphic representations of an already rich language. For example, children will listen to a story containing the grapheme "ea" (e.g., "a meal by the seaside," containing the words "beach," "sea," "seat," "meal," "peach," "cream," "tea,") can be listened to, and the listeners can hear and see (spelling) what is similar to these words. (This example is taken from http://www.bbc.co.uk/schools/words andpictures/longvow/poems/flash/ fpoem3.shtml) These activities imply moving away from an exclusive use of language for direct person-to-person communication: The activity requires thinking about how it sounds, not so much about

what it means. *Phonological awareness* is the term used to refer to the skill and understanding that spoken words are combinations of distinct sounds, which, in themselves, have no meaning. Writing words is (to a certain degree) a way of capturing a perceived sequence in these words. Phonological understanding is a rather abstract skill that is only mastered after sufficient exposure to and experience with spoken language. Are nonspeaking children at a disadvantage when it comes to recognize sounds and sound patterns? If so, can the disadvantage be compensated for by exercises in phonological coding? In a 1999 study, Foley and Pollatsek determined that participants with severe impaired and unintelligible speech could perform at normal levels for phonological coding of text. Card and Dodd (2006) compared speaking and nonspeaking children who had cerebral palsy on a number of phonological tasks. Although the two groups did not differ in all the tasks, there were differences in tasks for which an internalized articulatory loop could be used. In a study in which they trained three young AAC users in phoneme awareness, Truxler and O'Keefe (2007) were partially but not entirely successful, indicating that more and broader research is needed to determine critical and sufficient levels of phoneme awareness.

At the *initial reading* or *decoding stage*, the goal is to achieve effortless and automatic word recognition, a skill that good readers achieve in first grade. AAC users are often behind in this skill. Sturm, Spadorcia, Cunningham, Cali, Staples, and Erickson (2006) explore these and other stumbling blocks that seem to deprive children who are AAC users from critical literacy experiences. They suggest that the individualized educational and intervention plans for AAC users should explicitly include automatic word recognition activities.

In planning a literacy intervention program for children without functional speech, one needs to find alternatives for oral analytical skills. Educators often use activities that require "sounding out" words and listening to how they contrast or how they are similar (e.g., rhymes, alliterations). Sturm and colleagues suggest activities where words with minimal phonological or orthographic differences are displayed on one page of a device, and used in a variety of comparative exercises. Instead of oral manipulation of the words and their sounds, the AAC users are required to compare sounds and discover spelling similarities and differences.

LITERACY ACTIVITIES AS COMPENSATORY AAC STRATEGIES

Reading and writing, and all the activities that are related, are not just good supplements on top of AAC, they *are* in fact AAC! How can we ensure that we provide the right literacy intervention for children who are AAC users? Blischak (1995) discusses an individual approach that attempts to integrate literacy-specific skills into the educational planning of a child who has quadriplegic cerebral palsy and central vision impairment. The report highlights the possibilities of auditory scanning and the use of a Talking Screen (Words Plus Company). The author emphasizes that several factors probably converged in this case, with perhaps, most importantly, the language- and literacy-rich environment in which the child grew up (Blischak, 1995, p.18). The communication technique was an important gate

to literacy. And literacy, in turn, was the key to more independence and cognitive development. It should be noted that this was a report from the mid-1990s, more than 15 years ago. Since then, communication software has become more adaptive, and more efficient use is possible through word prediction and personalization. There is reason for optimism.

Educators and clinicians should take full advantage of AAC to provide and promote all possible literacy experiences and development. All too often, literacy is still not considered a priority goal for intervention. Smith (2005) proposes three key goals for literacy intervention for AAC users that fit within this perspective: (a) expand the literacy needs, (b) maximize the opportunities, and (c) minimize barriers to learning.

The first, expanding *the recognized literacy needs* starts with expectations. Reading and writing needs to become a high priority goal, hence time and efforts must be dedicated to pursue this. Regardless of age and reading level, it should be a goal to do *more*—more participation in a reading group, more reading materials to explore (in print or on the Internet), more pressure to use and depend on printed information and instructions. *Maximizing opportunities* implies "analysis of the daily routine and exploration of where additional or existing opportunities can be directed specifically to the needs of the target individual" (Smith, 2005, p. 185). Again, this means that "more" needs to be done, such as encouraging parents of young children to read more to them, suggesting that teachers of children at the emergent literacy level increase the number of literacy-based activities, while making sure that the AAC user is actively involved, and for adolescents to provide appealing skills and activities such as e-mail and text messaging. Finally, *minimizing barriers to learning* includes ensuring that the individual can obtain maximum visual access to print (large print may be required) or be given auditory help (activating recorded speech that reads all or part of the text). The importance of such a systematic literary focus is now broadly recognized. At the same time, the availability of good materials and well-thought-out individualized reading intervention plans remains an issue. It has been suggested that materials for assessment and intervention should be made available through the Internet to many (Iacono, 2004). Comparison of intervention results across languages and spelling systems can also help to understand how "deeper" phonological systems impact performance of learners, including AAC users (Dahlgren Sandberg et al., 2010; Erickson & Sachse, 2010).

MEASURING COMPETENCIES

Koppenhaver and colleagues (2009) explain that reading assessment in children who use AAC should be diagnostic and aim at the following three objectives: (1) developing reading profiles indicating learning strengths and weaknesses, (2) establishing instructional objectives, and (3) documenting reading growth over time (p. 87). In other words, the assessment should reveal a cognitive reading profile (that will be unique for each learner) as well as sufficient information for a measurable reading intervention plan.

Recent research, including comparative studies of children using different languages, shows that there is a large heterogeneity due to different cognitive, developmental, and linguistic profiles of

individual children (Dahlgren Sandberg et al., 2010). This is all the more reason to take individual skill assessment and observation of facilitating or hindering conditions seriously.

BECOMING A WRITER

Everybody can be a writer. There is not one child who is an AAC user who does not have an intriguing and appealing story to tell. Their experiences are sometimes sad, often uplifting, and occasionally heroic. It is important for them and for all educators to give them the tools to tell their stories.

However, writing proves to be an even bigger challenge than reading for many individuals who are AAC users. As is the case for expressive communication, the production of written text often is extremely slow and poses heavy requirements on short-term memory. Educators should not neglect this part of the curriculum. A systematic approach at the level of letter combination has been shown to give promising results (Millar, Light, & McNaughton, 2004). As is the case for reading, a writing assessment needs to be conducted. Given the complex nature of writing, such an assessment comprises the evaluation of prewriting skills (e.g., organizing the ideas to write about), composition skills, knowledge of spelling rules, grapho-motor abilities, and editing and revising skills (Foley, Koppenhaver, & Williams, 2009). Special attention needs to go to the use of assistive technology (e.g., aided communication devices) when constructing a written message. As discussed in other chapters of this book, the use of an aided method often requires special navigation skills, as well as short-term memory skills, and concentration due to slow production.

Despite the obvious challenges, there is an impressive number of skilled AAC users who are amazing writers. Some of them have published their own books or periodicals (some online). They can be (and are) an inspiration for young AAC users and their educators. One model and example is the Newsletter *Alternatively Speaking*, a periodical that has been entirely edited by AAC user Michael Williams. Another example is the book "Beneath the Surface," which contains literature contributions by 51 AAC users (Williams & Krezman, 2000).

AAC AND LITERACY IN THE FUTURE

The attention that literacy instruction and curricular adaption has received in the past two decades certainly matches its importance. A fascinating discussion and important research in the field of literacy skills by AAC users has emerged. This research and these developments are promising (Michael Barker, Saunders, & Brady, 2012).

POINTS TO REMEMBER

- The study of the relation between AAC and literacy is important because it can reveal something about how the lack of natural speech interacts with skills needed for reading and writing.
- Literacy skills can bring AAC users beyond the immediate needs and challenges of face-to-face communication.
- Literacy skills can be compensatory skills for AAC users.

- Experience with graphic AAC symbols can contribute to literacy acquisition by AAC users as long as educators take advantage of the possibilities of graphic symbols.
- Graphic symbol systems (more than symbol sets) share some structural similarities with orthographic systems because they have a sublexical system of graphic forms that are combined with each other.
- Educators must pursue a systematic and individualized intervention (and curriculum) that is geared to learning to read. Activities can include rapid word recognition, metalinguistic awareness training, rhyming games, and other alternatives for oral analytical exercises.
- Progress of literacy-related competencies needs to be measured and used to document and adjust an individualized literacy intervention plan.

REFERENCES

Blischak, D. M. (1995). Thomas the writer: Case study of a child with severe physical, speech, and visual impairments. *Language, Speech, and Hearing Services in Schools, 26*(1), 11–20.

Bondy, A. S., & Frost, L. A. (1994). The picture exchange communication system. *Focus on Autistic Behavior, 9*(3), 1–19.

Card, R., & Dodd, B. (2006). The phonological awareness abilities of children with cerebral palsy who do not speak. *AAC: Augmentative and Alternative Communication, 22*(3), 149–159.

Chall, J. (1983). *Stages of reading development.* New York, NY: McGraw-Hill.

Dahlgren Sandberg, A., Smith, M., & Larsson, M. (2010). An analysis of reading and spelling abilities of children using AAC: Understanding a continuum of competence. *AAC: Aug-*

mentative and Alternative Communication, 26(3), 191–202.

DeLoache, J., Pierroutsakos, S., & Troseth, G. (1996). The three R's of pictorial competence. In R. Vasta (Ed.), *Annals of child development* (Vol. 12, pp. 1–48). Bristol, PA: Jessica Kingsley.

DeLoache, J. S., Pierroutsakos, S. L., & Uttal, D. H. (2003). The origins of pictorial competence. *Current Directions in Psychological Science (Wiley-Blackwell), 12*(4), 114.

Erickson, K., & Clendon, S. (2009). Addressing the literacy demands of the curriculum for beginning readers and writers. In G. Soto & C. Zangari (Eds.), *Practically speaking: Language, literacy, and academic development for students with AAC needs* (pp. 195–215). Baltimore, MD: Paul H. Brookes.

Erickson, K., & Sachse, S. (2010). Reading acquisition, AAC and the transferability of English research to languages with more consistent or transparent orthographies. *AAC: Augmentative and Alternative Communication, 26*(3), 177–190.

Foley, B., Koppenhaver, D., & Williams, A. (2009). Writing assessment for students with AAC needs. In G. Soto & C. Zangari (Eds.), *Practically speaking: Language, literacy, and academic development for students with AAC needs* (pp. 93–128). Baltimore, MD: Paul H. Brookes.

Foley, B. E., & Pollatsek, A. (1999). Phonological processing and reading abilities in adolescents and adults with severe congenital speech impairments. *AAC: Augmentative & Alternative Communication, 15*(3), 156–173 (102 ref).

Iacono, T. A. (2004). Accessible reading intervention: A work in progress. *AAC: Augmentative and Alternative Communication, 20*(3), 179–190.

Justice, L. M., Skibbe, L., Canning, A., & Lankford, C. (2005). Pre-schoolers, print and storybooks: An observational study using eye movement analysis. *Journal of Research in Reading, 28*(3), 229–243.

Koppenhaver, D., Foley, B., & Williams, A. (2009). Diagnostic reading assessment for students with AAC needs. In G. Soto & C. Zangari (Eds.), *Practically speaking: Language, literacy, and academic development for students with AAC needs* (pp. 71–91). Baltimore, MD: Paul H. Brookes.

Light, J., & McNaughton, D. (2009). Addressing the literacy demands of the curriculum for conventional and more advanced readers and writers who require AAC. In G. Soto & C. Zangari (Eds.), *Practically speaking. Language, literacy, and academic development for students with AAC needs* (pp. 217–245). Baltimore, MD: Paul H. Brookes.

McNaughton, S., & Lindsay, P. (1995). Approaching literacy with AAC graphics. *AAC: Augmentative and Alternative Communication, 11*(4), 212–228.

Michael Barker, R., Saunders, K. J., & Brady, N. C. (2012). Reading instruction for children who use AAC: Considerations in the pursuit of generalizable results. *Augmentative and Alternative Communication, 28*(3), 160–170.

Millar, D. C., Light, J. C., & McNaughton, D. B. (2004). The effect of direct instruction and writer's workshop on the early writing skills of children who use augmentative and alternative communication. *AAC: Augmentative and Alternative Communication, 20*(3), 164–178.

Scherz, J., & Hart, P. (2002). Language, literacy, and AAC. *ASHA Leader, 7*(16), 17–18.

Smith, M. M. (2005). *Literacy and augmentative and alternative communication.* Burlington, MA: Elsevier Academic Press.

Sturm, J., Spadorcia, S. A., Cunningham, J. W., Cali, K. S., Staples, A., Erickson, K., Yoder, D., & Koppenhaver, D. A. (2006). What happens to reading between first and third grade? Implications for students who use AAC. *AAC: Augmentative and Alternative Communication, 22*(1), 21–36.

Truxler, J. E., & O'Keefe, B. M. (2007). The effects of phonological awareness instruction on beginning word recognition and spelling. *AAC: Augmentative and Alternative Communication, 23*(2), 164–176.

Van Balkom, H., & Verhoeven, L. (2010). Literacy learning in users of AAC: A neurocognitive perspective. *AAC: Augmentative and Alternative Communication, 26*(3), 149–157.

Williams, M., & Krezman, C. (Eds.). (2000). *Beneath the surface: Creative expressions of augmented communicators* (ISAAC Series: Vol. 2 ed.). Toronto, Canada: International Society for Augmentative and Alternative Communication.

CHAPTER 10

AAC and Natural Speech

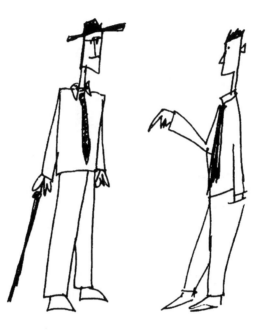

More than two hundred and fifty years ago in 1760, the French priest Charles-Michel de l'Epée started with the education of six deaf children in Paris. This endeavor rapidly developed into the first public school for deaf children, which is known today as the "Institut National de Jeunes Sourds" (National Institute of Young Deaf People). As a leading technique, De l'Epée used manual signs in a systematic way. He is remembered in the history of deaf education as the person who recognized the importance of manual signs for the education of deaf children. Already during his lifetime, de l'Epée encountered opposition to his idea that manual signing was a key solution to learn and to communicate for those who did not have access to spoken language because of deafness. In the 1770s, the German educator Heinicke had started to tutor and teach deaf children in Leipzig. Heinicke used a method suggested by the Swiss-Dutch physician Johan Amman who had taken up teaching speech to his deaf patients at the end of the 17th century, avoiding at all cost the use of manual signs. De l'Epée believed that manual signs were beneficial, whereas

Heinicke assumed manual signs would impede natural speech. Heinicke and De l'Epée wrote each other a series of letters, each one defending their own view on how to educate deaf children (Eriksson, 1998). This is one of the first and strongest examples of the controversy about the compatibility between expressive communicative modalities.

COMPATIBILITY AND INCOMPATIBILITY HYPOTHESES

This discussion that started from the beginning of public education for deaf children would continue through the 19th and 20th century into the present day. Few debates throughout the history of special education have stirred up as many emotions or have more divided individuals into vehemently opposing camps as this dispute. Why is that? One explanation is that this issue is much more than a mere difference of opinions about what would be the better method to teach deaf children. It touches on a deeper, underlying view about how the human mind works. It essentially comes down to assuming or rejecting the compatibility (or incompatibility) between modalities. Does manual signing prevent the development of speech—or, on the contrary, could it actually be beneficial for speech articulation? In other words, the question is whether the human mind has a tendency to limit primary language expression to one single modality (speech or sign), one sensory mode (visual or auditory), and one linguistic structure (spoken language grammar or sign language grammar), or whether no such limitations exist.

These opposing visions about the compatibility between natural speech and an alternative mode of communication have not remained limited to educational decisions in deaf education. A similar concern has risen in the field of AAC. Educators and parents often fear that the introduction of a nonspeech form of communication will be detrimental for the acquisition of the spoken language and especially of natural speech. In their 2005 article, Romski and Sevcik characterize this fear as one of the five stubborn myths about AAC.

THE INCOMPATIBILITY HYPOTHESIS

What exactly are the concerns of those who believe the use of AAC might have a negative impact on natural speech and language use? The following underlying issues and assumptions are at the core of the issue:

1. The use of AAC could lead to less overall effort by the user as he or she may lose the drive and the motivation to communicate through natural speech (a slightly different variant of this view states that educators and clinicians may give up efforts toward training of speech once alternative modalities have been introduced);.

2. The use of AAC will lead to the creation of messages that structurally deviate from English (or whichever the spoken language is that is used in the environment of the person).

The debate deliberates: (a) a view on the compatibility between natural speech and the nonspeech modalities: is there a mutual inhibitory effect, a facilitation effect, or none of the above? (b) a view on transmodal interference: will the syntactical structure of one modality (e.g., manual signing) be transposed to the syntactical structure of English (or the spoken language of the user)? (c) a view on total mental lexical storage capacity across modalities, and (d) a view on the motivational effects of the use of one modality toward the other (will effective communication in one modality encourage or discourage the user to make efforts in the speech modality?). There are few direct answers to give to these questions, but some clues may come from the existing knowledge on bilingualism, multimodality, and motivation toward the use of communication modalities.

INFORMATION FROM BILINGUALISM

The discussion about compatibility of modalities is somehow linked to the hypothesis of limitations in human linguistic competence, that is, the suggestion that more than one modality is too much to process. However, the study of bilingualism indicates that the human linguistic potential is impressive. What is the linguistic-communicative capacity of humans? Interestingly, one hardly finds any estimates in literature. However, one can find interesting accounts of individuals who know an unusual number of languages. For example, the lexicographer Noah Webster reportedly knew more than 20 languages. How exceptional is that? Maybe less than we tend to think. In the summer of 2009, I taught a course, "Multicultural Communication," to a group of health care and educational workers from different countries in Africa and Asia. The course was taught in English although none of the participants (nor

the instructor, being me) was a native speaker of English. The 18 students were from Burundi, the Democratic Republic of Congo, India, Indonesia, Pakistan, the Philippines, Rwanda, and Vietnam. I already knew that in most regions of the world, monolingualism (the use of one language) is rather the exception than the rule. In many areas of the world, people switch from language to language all the time. I decided that we could conduct a little survey on ourselves, how many languages did we know? All of the participants reported that they knew and used more than three languages. Some possessed more than eight languages. For example, take Simon, a 36-year-old administrator in a psychiatric hospital in the Democratic Republic of Congo. His first language was Kiyombe, which he acquired from his mother. However, this was only the beginning of his many language acquisitions. He heard and learned to communicate in Kikongo from the age of two and in Lingala from the age of three, both languages being spoken by members of his extended family (living in or near his home). At age 8, he started to learn and use French, which was one of the instructional languages used in school. At the age of 15, when he entered high school, he started to learn and use English. All the while, interacting with members from other tribes and villages, he learned Kintandu, Kimanianga, and Kimbona. At the age of 28, he also picked up Tshiluba. To Westerners who often do not master more than two or at most three languages, this may appear exceptional and maybe at the brink of what we are cognitively able to store and process. However, in the same group of 18 students in my 2009 course, the average number of languages known was five! Language proficiency or mastery of English was not a requirement to be a student in this group. There is no reason to believe that these participants would not be representative for the language mastery of young educated individuals in developing areas of the world.

In other words, one does not need to be exceptionally gifted to be able to learn and use different languages. Does that observation extend to the mastery of different modalities? If most people have the capacity to learn several languages, maybe this is an indication that the average person does have the potential to acquire several linguistic systems.

MULTIMODALITY

There are many obvious examples that demonstrate that modalities can be compatible and mutually reinforcing. The most obvious examples are: speaking and writing, and listening and reading. If modalities would be incompatible, it would—in its strictest form—mean that individuals who learn to read and write would lose some of their speaking skills. This hypothesis, of course, is so absurd that no researcher has looked into it; people who are good with the pen (or the computer) are generally also good with speaking. Modalities appear to reinforce each other. Or, what is more likely, speaking and writing are the expressions of the same underlying language mastery (Berninger et al., 2006). By practicing speech, we strengthen our language skills from which writing will benefit, and vice versa; by practicing writing we reinforce the underlying language that is the underpinning of speech.

Could the same be true for other modalities? Would manual signing strengthen underlying language skills and thus be beneficial for speech? Maybe this may be too much of a leap in our thinking since the underlying language structures for manual signing are different than those for spoken language? What about the use of a speech-generating device? Would that facilitate natural speech? It can be the basis for future research.

SPEECH AND GESTURE

Before addressing these questions, let us look at another body of research that could be informative for us, the relationship between *speech and gesture*. In the past 30 years, an impressive number of studies have been conducted that explore how gesturing, language, and speech are connected and how they are mutually supportive (or inhibitory). Most of the studies have focused on natural gestures. McNeill (1992, 2000, 2005) and his collaborators analyzed hours of natural gesture production that spontaneously occurs along with spontaneous speech. In McNeill's account, speech and gesture are in a dynamic relation with each other, both emerging from the same underlying message. Gestures often capture the more imagistic characteristics of the message (spreading the arms to indicate "big") while speech contains more the analytic information. In McNeill's view, gesture and speech are two sides of the same process (see also Chapter 4).

A number of theories in evolutionary linguistics state that gestures predate speech, or, that gestures have functioned as an intrinsic element in the chain of evolution of the homo sapiens from a nonspeaking to a speaking species (Corballis, 2008). The first symbols in communication between humans, according to these accounts, would have been gestural, and somehow must have led, in a continuous or discontinuous way, to the development of speech. Speech, according to many present-day psycholinguists (e.g., Levelt, 1993), is the coordinated production of articulatory gestures, each one roughly corresponding to a syllable. Of course, one must resist the overinterpretation of drawing parallels between evolutionary pathways from gesture to speech and the development of children from early gestural communication (in the prelinguistic stage) to the early speech communication.

Since the 1980s, psycholinguists and cognitive psychologists have paid special attention to the possibility that natural gestures could have a facilitating effect on speech. Hundreds of articles have been published focusing on some of the aspects of the relationships between *gesture and speech* and *gesture and language*. A wealth of studies and observations give support to McNeill's view that gesture and speech are not just compatible, but that they are intimately internally linked.

Gesture and Aphasia

For decades, it has been noted that the spontaneous gesturing of individuals with aphasia somehow reflects the nature of their spoken language production. Lemay, David, and Thomas (1988) reported that patients with Broca's aphasia would gesture more with "beats" ("baton-like") and pointing, while those with Wernicke's aphasia would display more "kinetographs" (gestures that depict movements). These authors agree with the view that gesture and speech both originate from one central mental organizer. Raymer (2007) reports on intervention with *indi-viduals with aphasia* in whom gesture appears to facilitate word finding. Other studies suggest the same or similar results (Marshall, 2006) as those mentioned by Raymer in her report. Marshall critically analyzes the results and suggests that it is not just any gesture that will do the job of helping a person with aphasia activate expression of words and phrases. What seems to matter is that the gestures have a "language-like" character. They have to contain meaning, either as lexical elements (e.g., gestures with a conventional meaning), which would allow them to map on a word, or as the equivalent of a phrase. Kara Morgenstern, one of my students in 2009 and 2010, taught Bonvillian's simplified signs (see Chapter 4) to individuals with anomia. Her results provided evidence for the hypothesis that "naming skills for targeted words can be improved following treatment (semantic, phonological, gestural) for some individuals with anomia" (Morgenstern, Braddock, Bonvillian, Steele, & Loncke, 2009). Similar results have been found for people with fluency problems. Mayberry, Jaques, and DeDe (1998) analyzed transcription of videotapes of stutterers and noticed an almost synchronized pattern of stuttered speech and the way gestures were made.

Gesture and Second Language Learning

There are even some suggestions that one can use gesturing in learning words from *foreign languages*. Allen (1995) conducted a learning experiment with students studying French as a foreign language. She paired French words with "emblematic" gestures and found that the participants who were exposed to the linked condition performed better than those who were in the control group. In a similar experiment,

Kelly, McDevitt, and Esch (2009) found that novel Japanese words were easier and faster to learn if the words were presented together with hand gestures. Further research by Kelly and his collaborators (Kelly, Creigh, & Bartolotti, 2010) suggest the formation of neuropsychological integrated networks underlying these word-gesture connections, facilitating word retrieval in both word production and word recognition.

TESTING THE MULTIMODALITY HYPOTHESIS

A similar line of thinking was the basis of two studies that Loncke and his associates (2008, 2009) conducted with undergraduate college students. Their purpose was to "test the multimodality hypothesis." In the first study they looked at the effect of added auditory feedback to the process of learning pseudowords. While there was no difference in learning results for the auditory feedback condition in words with a simple phonological structure (words with two syllables), the auditory feedback did matter when the words were more complex (three or four syllables). In the second experiment, the authors added gestures to the mix. They used symbolic gestures borrowed from Bonvillian's Simplified Sign System, and "phonological gestures" that were constructed with hand alphabet configurations combined with a movement representing the syllabic structure (a rhythmical movement with a "beat" for each syllable). The results showed again a superior performance for the condition with the added symbolic (simplified, iconic) sign, but not for the phonological gesture. Today's research appears to indicate that representational

gestures do indeed facilitate speech (e.g., Kita & Davies, 2009). It appears that gesturing has the potential to facilitate the use and development of speech, especially the word finding aspect of speech. More specifically, gestures may help in lexical searches (finding the words in your mental lexicon) and in initiating the motor programs needed for speech.

Hubbard, Wilson, Callan, and Dapretto (2009) report on a study in which they used functional magnetic resonance imaging (fMRI) investigating how persons perceived speech that was accompanied by "beat" gestures. McNeill defines beat gestures (1992) as rhythmical movements that go along with the pulsation of speech (p. 15; see Chapter 4). These gestures have no symbolic meaning as such, except that they represent some sequential structure of syllables, words, or phrases. Hubbard and her coauthors found that the bilateral nonprimary auditory cortex showed greater activity when speech was accompanied by a beat gesture than in instances where speech was presented alone. This data, the authors conclude, suggest a common neural substrate for processing speech and gesture, which gives neuropsychological support to the behavioral description of speech and gesture working together.

TRANSMODAL INTERFERENCE

Will the syntactical structure of one modality (e.g., manual signing) be transposed to the syntactical structure of English (or the spoken language of the user)?

The phenomenon of *interference* has been widely described and documented in research on bilingualism. A French-English bilingual person may erroneously say, "I have 35 years," which is a direct structural translation from the French, "j'ai trente cinq ans." Most bilingual speakers, however, are good at keeping the two systems separated so that "language mixing" or "code mixing" is a relatively infrequent phenomenon. The most accepted hypothesis is that the two languages are stored in the mental system in such a way that one can remain inactive while the other is being activated. For example, a bilingual Spanish-English speaker puts her Spanish to sleep while she speaks English. How is this done? It is generally believed that a speaker is sensitive to cues in the environment, which activate an internal switch for one specific language. The assumption is that, while a person acquires a second language (or two languages at the same time), he or she builds internally distinct linguistic networks. *Code switching*, the phenomenon that bilingual speakers automatically can switch back and forth, is one indication that language systems are neurolinguistically separately marked (Grosjean, 2012).

But does this also apply to AAC? That is less certain. A typical bilingual speaker is usually in an either-or situation: you speak language A or language B, not the two at the same time. The multimodality situation in which AAC users find themselves is different; they are expected to respond to English natural speakers through a variety of codes and non-English elements. If a natural English speaker asks a communication board user, "tell me what you did during the weekend," the user may activate the graphic symbols "play," "I," "Jerry" (the name of his little brother) to indicate that he and his brother have played together. The word order is clearly not English (that would be "I-play-Jerry"). In such a case, it could be argued that the visual-graphic nature

of the graphic symbols suggests the user to use a non-English order (in this—fictitious—example) despite the fact that the interlocutor started in English. There is little research on what this potential structural incompatibility does to the acquisition of the structures of the spoken language. Therapists will often train the AAC user to follow the English order when they are combining symbols. One intervention goal would be to "use the symbols in the English order." But is that a reasonable expectation? Could it be that we are forcing graphic-visual message construction in an unnatural English-type order? Therapists may encourage the "use of the symbols in the right/correct order." Besides the fact that this implies a value judgment on the utterance of the client (is a non-English type utterance really "not correct"?), we do not really know what exactly intervention should consist of and what the effects of intervention would be.

LEXICAL STORAGE CAPACITY ACROSS MODALITIES

When asking average language users how many words they think they know, one usually obtains an underestimation of what their real knowledge probably is. The first time a person hears that average language users know tens of thousands of words, they are typically astonished! What does this tell us? Although humans use language all the time, their reflective knowledge of how the system actually works is limited (unless they took a linguistics or a psycholinguistics course). Therefore, a statement on the "capacity" to have and know words, graphic symbols, manual signs, or other symbols might be more based on an intuition than on actual knowledge. Hence, we should be careful with statements like, "let's not confuse our student by adding more graphic symbols or more signs to what he already knows." We simply don't know enough about how much word/lexical learning capacity there is.

MOTIVATIONAL ASPECTS

Does the introduction of accessible modalities lead to a decrease of motivation to use and practice the "harder" modality, i.e., speech? Does the principle of "the law of the least effort" apply to the use of AAC? The law of least effort would predict that the introduction of a "more accessible" modality (because it is more within reach for the person's developmental, cognitive, or motor level) will keep a person from doing the extra efforts to learn the "harder" modalities.

No doubt that this is the explanation why, traditionally, AAC was often only introduced to a child after all other "more normal" options were exhausted. In many practices, even today, AAC is considered to be a last resort. Introducing AAC before everything else would have been tried and failed, would be an indication that one gives up natural speech prematurely.

But is this the right approach? In the first place, it needs mentioning that typical development always goes from the more accessible to the more complex. The reason why gestural communication is prominent in typically developing children between ages 18 and 24 months is precisely that: in a period that natural articulated and coordinated speech is still neuromotorically difficult, normal children augment their communication with gestures. Does the use of gestures in normal children delay the development of speech, or does it have a negative influence? It does not! At present, most scholars agree that in normal development, there is a sequential stage development from: (1) expressing symbolic skills in a nonvocal way, over (2) a "bimodal period" (Volterra, Caselli, Capirci, & Pizzuto, 2005) around the age of 14 months where gesture and vocal utterances coexist, to (3) a predominantly vocal expressive way. Gesture development appears to be more a launching pad than a hindrance for speech in normal development.

The data also suggest that there are natural-spontaneous forms of augmentative communication that advance the child's development in case of neurological problems. Sauer, Levine, and Goldin-Meadow (2010) found that children with brain injuries, who were spontaneously using more gestures at the age of 18 months, were less likely to have a language delay. Those who had been limited gesturers, turned out to have a language delay.

The lack of or the delayed development of spontaneous gestures can thus in itself be an indication of language and communication problems. Sowden, Perkins, and Cleggs (2008) looked at the use of gesture in children with a diagnosis on the autism spectrum. Their case studies suggest that developmental delays co-occur in both speech and gesture use.

The observations of the use of gesture do not give reason to believe that the "law of the least effort" works here. If that were the case, typical gesturing children would not develop speech or develop it at a much slower rate, and later. On the contrary, something else is going on here. It appears that the use of nonspeech forms drives normal children to further explore modalities of symbolic expression, leading them to the discovery of speech.

These studies give us reason to believe that: (1) the use of "alternative" communication forms to speech are a natural phenomenon as shown by normally developing children who go through a gesturing period (prior to the age of 14 months) before fully developing speech, (2) the use of alternative modes may help the communicator build an internal substrate that will support both speech and nonspeech modalities, and (3) nonspeech communication forms may motivate the communicator to explore more complex communication forms (speech).

AAC EVIDENCE

How certain can we be that this reasoning applies to AAC? What is the evidence? Millar, Light, and Schlosser (2006) conducted a research review of studies that mentioned effects on speech of some form of AAC. They reviewed the literature and identified 23 studies providing data on 67 individuals. Most of the cases were individuals with intellectual disabilities or an autism-related developmental disorder. The AAC intervention in most cases consisted of the use of manual signing or low-tech communication. Unfortunately, a majority of these clinical studies establish sufficient experimental control, which forced the authors to zoom in on six studies describing the results of 27 cases. Interestingly, none of the cases showed a decrease in natural speech. In 11% of the cases, no effect of the AAC intervention for speech was reported. An impressive majority of 89% showed some improvement in natural speech. The authors con-

cluded "we have moved from an inconclusive to a suggestive relationship between natural speech output and AAC."

Schlosser and Wendt (2008) did similar work focusing on studies with children diagnosed with autism. They looked at nine single-subject experimental design and two group studies. Analysis of these data led the authors to conclude, "There is no evidence that AAC intervention hinders speech production in children with autism or PDD-NOS (Pervasive Developmental Disorder—Not otherwise specified)." However, the results of most studies show that the gains are limited. Spectacular development of speech is rather rare. How can this be explained? The authors point to a possible "ceiling effect," cases where the participant scored the maximum outcome and where improvement (on the test) was simply not measurable. There may also be other factors at work. One could, again, be related to the stimulation and the expectations that caregivers, educators, and therapists may have. Maybe AAC does not hinder speech, but it may also be naïve (and unwarranted) to expect that speech will emerge automatically, as a side effect of introducing AAC. We need more reflection and more research on how we should connect the communicative objectives, the language objectives, and the speech objectives in our interventions.

Instead of just looking at the effects of AAC for speech, we may want to be more proactive and search for the use of AAC specifically to promote speech development. Some studies go in that direction. For example, Cumley and Swanson (1999) explored the possibility that the use of AAC would be helpful in the development of speech patterns for children who were diagnosed with apraxia of speech.

THE EFFECTS OF DEVICE-GENERATED SPEECH

In the previous paragraphs, we have mainly talked about the effects of manual signing, gestures, and low-tech communication intervention, without mentioning speech that is generated by a device. What about that? Could it be that speech-generating devices do facilitate natural speech? Or can one argue exactly the opposite (i.e., that the use of device speech somehow takes away the need to develop an internal phonology that is underlying natural speech?). On the one hand, a case can be made that the use of a speech-generating device can have an effect on the development of an internal phonology, which, in turn, can be a driving force for the development of speech skills. Blischak (1999) pointed out that the development of phonological awareness should be a priority for research and intervention. Phonological awareness is a central component for the development of literacy—a set of skills that is, unfortunately, often underdeveloped in AAC users (most likely through a combination of lack of expectations, experiences, and inadequate intervention). Will speech-generating devices help in the development of an internal phonology? Blischak, Lombardino, and Dyson (2003) provide some explanations why there could be a positive impact from the use of speech-generating devices on the development of natural speech. These include: (1) the consistency of the synthetic speech output, (2) reinforcement (each time the speech output is activated, the mental representation by the user is reinforced), (3) strengthening of the phonological code of the words, and (4) multimodality: through the device, the user can link a graphic symbol, a printed word, an acoustic output with a motor-articulatory representation (i.e., or one would actually speak). Artificial speech can lead to natural speech.

Throughout this chapter, it has become clear that more research needs to be done. Research should focus on what the effects of AAC are on speech (and other functions). We need to understand better how multimodality works so that we can replace our "beliefs" ("I think AAC is good for speech," "No, I don't think so, etc.") with supportive evidence. In the end, it can give us fascinating information that transcends the field of AAC as an applied field. It can tell us something about how the human mind works with symbols and how it connects their modalities.

NATURAL SPEECH AS A GOAL OR A PREFERENCE

We will need to find the best ways to address the daily challenges that are connected with this issue. Despite all the successes that we may have with AAC, success is always codetermined by our perception of what the goals, the aspirations, and the dreams are. In their 2004 study of AAC using children in Mexican-American families, McCord and Soto quote the mother of a teenager who is the most proficient AAC user in the group:

Mother: "What I want more now than anything is for her to be able to talk. She can talk a little, 'mama,' 'papi,' 'Laura,' 'Hugo,' 'Tonio.' She can say a few words, 'comer' (eat), 'vamanos' (let's go), various words like that she can say."

Researcher: "How about with the DeltaTalker? What do you think of her using that to talk?"

Mother: "Well no, the machine is not a good apparatus for communicating with us. I prefer that she use her voice and her signs to communicate with us. But the machine, that's of no use for talking." (p. 217)

These examples illustrate how important it is that the alternative modes are valued by the user as well as by the communication partners.

CONCLUSION

Theoretical evidence points in the direction that modalities exert a mutual positive and reinforcing influence. Internalized modality representations are interconnected. Activation of alternative modalities increases the activation of speech, if speech is paired and associated with the alternative modes. Clinical evidence supports this compatibility hypothesis. Natural speech does not suffer from the use of alternative modes. On the contrary, the introduction of the alternative modes can offer a renewed avenue in the pursuit of speech goals.

POINTS TO REMEMBER

- The incompatibility hypothesis suggests that negative or interfering effects limit the development of natural speech once alternative modalities are introduced.

- The compatibility hypothesis suggests that internal mental representations of modalities are part of a network that can have a reinforcing effect on speech.
- Similarities between multilingualism and multimodality can give us clues to understand the capacity to master communication in different modalities.
- Gesture studies indicate that there is a natural supportive link between gesture use and speech.
- Clinical case and group studies point to a suggestive positive relationship between natural speech output and AAC.

REFERENCES

Allen, L. Q. (1995). The effects of emblematic gestures on the development and access of mental representations of French expressions. *Modern Language Journal, 79*(4), 521–529.

Amman, J. C. (n.d.). *The talking deaf.* [Surdus loquens.] Available from http://www.guten berg.org/ebooks/13014

Berninger, V. W., Abbott, R. D., Jones, J., Wolf, B. J., Gould, L., Anderson-Youngstrom, M., & Apel, K. (2006). Early development of language by hand: Composing, reading, listening, and speaking connections; Three letter-writing modes; and fast mapping in spelling. *Developmental Neuropsychology, 29*(1), 61–92.

Blischak, D. M. (1999). Increases in natural speech production following experience with synthetic speech. *Journal of Special Education Technology, 14*(2), 44–53.

Blischak, D. M., Lombardino, L. J., & Dyson, A. T. (2003). Use of speech-generating devices: In support of natural speech. *AAC: Augmentative and Alternative Communication, 19*(1), 29–35.

Corballis, M. (2008). Time on our hands: How gesture and the understanding of the past and future helped shape language. *Behavioral and Brain Sciences, 31*(5), 517–517.

Cumley, G. D., & Swanson, S. (1999). Augmentative and alternative communication options for children with developmental apraxia of speech: Three case studies. *AAC: Augmentative and Alternative Communication, 15*(2), 110–125.

Eriksson, P. (1998). *The history of deaf people*. Orebro, Sweden: National Swedish Agency for Special Education.

Grosjean, F. (2012). An attempt to isolate, and then differentiate, transfer and interference. *International Journal of Bilingualism, 16*(1), 11–21.

Hubbard, A. L., Wilson, S. M., Callan, D. E., & Dapretto, M. (2009). Giving speech a hand: Gesture modulates activity in auditory cortex during speech perception. *Human Brain Mapping, 30*(3), 1028–1037.

Kelly, S. D., Creigh, P., & Bartolotti, J. (2010). Integrating speech and iconic gestures in a stroop-like task: Evidence for automatic processing. *Journal of Cognitive Neuroscience, 22*(4), 683–694.

Kelly, S. D., McDevitt, T., & Esch, M. (2009). Brief training with co-speech gesture lends a hand to word learning in a foreign language. *Language and Cognitive Processes, 24*(2), 313–334.

Kita, S., & Davies, T. S. (2009). Competing conceptual representations trigger co-speech representational gestures. *Language and Cognitive Processes, 24*(5), 761–775.

LeMay, A., David, R., & Thomas, A. P. (1988). The use of spontaneous gesture by aphasic patients. *Aphasiology, 2*, 137–145.

Levelt, W. J. M. (1993). *Speaking: From intention to articulation* (1st MIT Pbk. ed.). Cambridge, MA: MIT Press.

Loncke, F., Crato, D., Canty, T., Goldkamp, J., Leconte, C., & Marichez, D. (2008). *Are users of speech-generating devices using an internal phonology?* Presentation at the Annual Convention of the American Speech-Language and Hearing Association, Chicago, IL.

Loncke, F., Hilton, J., Weng, P., & Corthals, P. (2009). *Testing the multimodality hypothesis. Learning printed words with and without auditory and gesture feedback*. Presentation at the 3rd Annual Conference for Clinical Augmentative and Alternative Communication, Pittsburgh, PA.

Luria, A. R. (1970). *Traumatic aphasia*. The Hague, the Netherlands: Mouton.

Marshall, J. (2006). The role of gesture in aphasia therapy. *Advances in Speech Language Pathology, 8*(2), 110–114.

Mayberry, R. I., Jaques, J., & DeDe, G. (1998). What stuttering reveals about the development of the gesture-speech relationship. *New Directions for Child Development, (79)*, 77–87.

McCord, M. S., & Soto, G. (2004). Perceptions of AAC: An ethnographic investigation of Mexican-American families. *AAC: Augmentative and Alternative Communication, 20*(4), 209–27.

McNeill, D. (1992). *Hand and mind: What gestures reveal about thought*. Chicago, IL: University of Chicago Press.

McNeill, D. (2000). *Language and gesture*. Cambridge, UK: Cambridge University Press.

McNeill, D. (2005). *Gesture and thought*. Chicago, IL: University of Chicago Press.

Millar, D. C., Light, J. C., & Schlosser, R. W. (2006). The impact of augmentative and alternative communication intervention on the speech production of individuals with developmental disabilities: A research review. *Journal of Speech, Language, and Hearing Research, 49*(2), 248–264.

Morgenstern, K., Braddock, B., Bonvillian, J., Steele, R., & Loncke, F. (2009). *Verbal and simplified sign system treatments in adults with acquired anomia of speech*. Presentation at the 3rd Annual Conference for Clinical Augmentative and Alternative Communication, Pittsburgh, PA.

Raymer, A. M. (2007). Gestures and words: Facilitating recovery in aphasia. *The ASHA Leader, 12*(8), 8–11.

Romski, M., & Sevcik, R. A. (2005). Augmentative communication and early intervention: Myths and realities. *Infants & Young Children, 18*(3), 174–185.

Sauer, E., Levine, S. C., & Goldin-Meadow, S. (2010). Early gesture predicts language delay in children with pre- or perinatal brain lesions. *Child Development, 81*(2), 528–539.

Schlosser, R. W., & Wendt, O. (2008). Effects of augmentative and alternative communication intervention on speech production in children with autism: A systematic review. *American Journal of Speech-Language Pathology, 17*(3), 212–230.

Sowden, H., Perkins, M., & Cleggs, J. (2008). The co-development of speech and gesture in children with autism. *Clinical Linguistics & Phonetics, 22*(10 & 11), 804–813.

Volterra, V., Caselli, C., Capirci, O., & Pizzuto, E. (2005). Gesture and the emergence and development of language. In M. Tomasello & D. Slobin (Eds.), *Beyond nature—Nurture. Essays in honor of Elizabeth Bates* (pp. 3–40). Mahwah, NJ: Lawrence Erlbaum Associates.

CHAPTER 11

AAC and Assessment

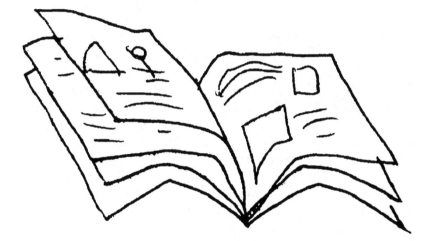

The purpose of assessment in AAC is the determination *if* a person can benefit from AAC intervention, *what* AAC intervention should consist of, and what the *predictions* for functioning would be. AAC assessment distinguishes itself from diagnostics of the primary cause of the language or communication disorder. These diagnoses include both developmental (e.g., Autism Spectrum Disorder, Down syndrome) and acquired disorders (e.g., aphasia, ALS). However, such a diagnosis *in itself* is not a motivation for the use of AAC. Within these medical and neurodevelopmental conditions, there is a continuum from no or low need to high need for AAC support. If there are indications that an individual could benefit from AAC, the assessment will need to determine the appropriate and optimal nature of AAC intervention for the client.

AAC ASSESSMENT IS PART OF AAC INTERVENTION

From the very moment AAC is considered to be a potential help for a person, assessment and intervention become interconnected. In many cases, AAC assessment is not a one-time event but an ongoing process: the observed needs by the potential AAC clients and their communication partners lead to questions about and requests for solutions, which are attempted to be met by the assessment. Once outcomes of the assessment are implemented, the results should be evaluated against what was projected and predicted. The effects of AAC implementation can lead to adjustments in how AAC is used by a specific client. The effects of AAC implementation can also put in motion new developments in a person's life (e.g., new social contacts, ways to ask questions, etc.). For example, AAC can help in opening academic avenues for a person which, in turn, can help a person to explore career opportunities.

DETERMINATION OF AAC NEEDS

As discussed in previous chapters (especially Chapter 2), AAC is an umbrella term for a range of activities, solutions, and strategies that make communication possible or more effective for individuals who have limitations in the use of natural and functional speech. The need for AAC can stem from quite different physical or mental etiologies, and the solutions will, accordingly, be different.

"Communication skills" is a theoretical construct. We like to describe it as a set of mental and human abilities, which can be analyzed and measured as separate components. We will need to gain a good understanding of: (1) how the different abilities interact, and (2) how strong their relative importance is for a person's communication. For example, do "vocabulary" and "memory" carry the same weight when it comes to predicting AAC outcomes?

The framework, based on Levelt's blueprint for the speaker, which we have used in previous chapters, can again serve us as guidance for when we focus on assessments of AAC needs and inter-

vention solutions. When looking at the different implicit operations involved in natural speech production (or online communication expression) one can easily see that different types of skills are at play.

Each time we conduct an AAC assessment, we implicitly use a construct of what AAC entails. Already from the moment that we plan the assessment, we think of different components: cognitive, linguistic, motor, perceptual, and social-pragmatic skills (Figure 11–1). When assessing the strengths and weaknesses of a person for the use of some form of AAC, the relative weight of these components will need to be addressed.

Cognitive operations are at play in conceiving the intention of the utterance and identifying the elements to be communicated. They are also important in interpreting all information that pertains to deciding the relevance of messages received (Sperber & Wilson, 1986). *Linguistic operations* include the lexical searches (and the navigations to find the symbols) and the way the message is planned as a sequence of symbols, manual signs. *Motor operations* are the actual behaviors that the person executes in order to produce the message in a perceivable way. This includes speech articulation, the actual performance of manual signs, and the behaviors needed to operate a communication aid. *Perceptual operations* are active when a message is decoded. In order for communication to be successful, one must be able to process the auditory, visual, or tactual information that contains the message. For most individuals, hearing and seeing are the senses with which communicative signals are perceived. Therefore, auditory and visual testing will provide essential information. For potential AAC users, there are additional reasons to pay

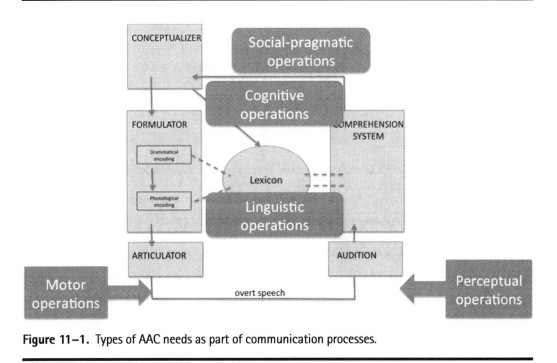

Figure 11–1. Types of AAC needs as part of communication processes.

sufficient attention to this matter. First, many AAC candidates are at risk for perceptual impairments. Second, many of the AAC solutions use visual information (manual signs, graphic symbols, computer or device displays, and keyboards). And *third*, it should be remembered that *recognition* of speech, manual signs, and graphic symbols relies on more than just sensory acuity. It requires the potential to recognize patterns, an ability that may be impaired in children with severe developmental limitations and in adults with acquired neurological dysfunctions. For example we might encounter cases of *visual* or *auditory agnosia*, a limitation in recognizing what is heard or seen. Depending on the background of the client, a neuropsychological examination may be recommended. *Social-pragmatic operations* are those that connect the messages with social contexts and understanding

of other people's knowledge. The latter is often called *theory of mind* (Frith & Frith, 2005).

COMMUNICATIVE COMPETENCE AS OBJECT OF ASSESSMENT

AAC assessment is an exploration of the potential of a person to develop communicative competence. The abovementioned groups of skills are building blocks of this competence. Light (1989) proposed to break down the rather general term "communicative competence" into four different competencies—a way of characterizing and differentiating individual AAC components. *Linguistic competence* refers to the linguistic skills a person employs in communication. It includes the knowledge of words, lexical access, and mastery of combinatorial-syntactic rules. *Operational competence* is the ability of a person to execute mental and motor functions as part of action planning within AAC. This can include the operation of a device (including navigation, switch use, and memorizing the sequence of steps), the physical execution of a manual sign, and the ability to manipulate graphic symbol communication cards. *Social competence* refers to the person's set of skills that allows him or her to take and maintain a place in the social context, making and maintaining friendships, and establishing rapport. *Strategic competence* involves being able to make the best of the often limited means you have. It includes specific pragmatic skills such as being able to work around the problem of speed limitations of the device. Or, to put it simply, strategic competence is about the ability of getting things done despite the communication limitations.

action. Is interaction merely limited to repetitive routines in which the AAC user and the partner repeatedly do the same thing? Does the AAC user have opportunities to exert a range of pragmatic functions such as requesting, rejecting, asking questions, and making comments? Does the AAC user initiate or merely react to exchanges that have been initiated by others? Third, the *material components* are the tools that are available to facilitate communication. These include all the assistive nontech and tech devices that can be part of AAC (e.g., graphic symbols, communication boards, speech generating devices, nondedicated tools).

An attempt to characterize the total "basket" of factors that can lead to AAC success is represented in Figure 11–2. All of these factors need to be considered to obtain a full picture when planning, conducting, and interpreting an AAC assessment.

ASSESSMENT OF THE LARGER PICTURE

Focusing on the communication process solely will not yield a complete picture of what determines whether AAC can be successful. The *communication partners* constitute another important factor: their habits, expectations, style, patience, and ability (e.g., operational knowledge of the device, knowledge of the manual sign system), and willingness to invest efforts and time in the interaction can have an enormous influence on the quality and intensity of communication. Second, much depends on *interactive components*. These include the time and the opportunities for interaction and information exchange, as well as the quality and content of the inter-

PRINCIPLES OF AAC ASSESSMENT

The purpose of an AAC assessment is to determine which modifications in the ways of communicating by person are likely to bring important improvements in effectiveness and quality of communication. Underlying to this purpose are a number of implicit views:

1. Assessment of present behavior and skills needs to be interpreted in terms of functionality;
2. Observation of today's behavior and skills will provide information on the possibilities to acquire new behaviors and new skills;
3. Communicative behavior is measurable; and

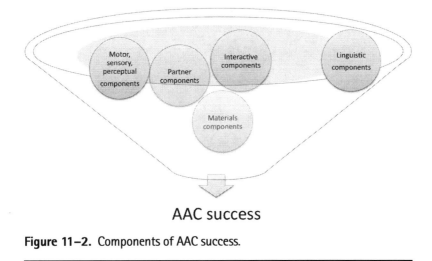

AAC success

Figure 11–2. Components of AAC success.

4. AAC is partially measurable through the assessment of language components such as vocabulary.

1. Assessment of Present Behavior and Skills Needs to Be Interpreted in Terms of Functionality

The purpose of AAC is functional: AAC has its legitimacy as long as it allows people to function better in their environment, because it intends to provide them with new, better, and more effective ways to connect with others. The International Classification of Functioning (ICF) (Rosenbaum & Stewart, 2004) constitutes a framework for improving people's quality of life (at all ages) through measurable interventions. The central concept in the ICF approach is the importance of participation in social life. Participation is reflected in the potential to perform activities as a result of an interaction of "body structure and function" with personal and environmental factors (Figure 11–3).

This framework nicely fits AAC. AAC performance is *not* a direct predictable outcome of body structure or functioning (be it that these are the source or reason why an AAC solution is sought), but it depends on the interplay of all the factors (personal factors, environmental challenges, coaching, opportunities, as well as critical activities; Murphy & Boa, 2012). Recently, there have been promising attempts to apply this framework directly to AAC in children (Rowland et al., 2012; see also http://www.icfcy.org/aac#ui-tabs-1).

2. Observation of Today's Behavior and Skills Will Provide Information on the Possibilities to Acquire New Behaviors and New Skills

Assessment consists of a series of observations (tests, tasks, questionnaires) that are interpreted in light of what is known about the person's background (physical and psychological condition, educational

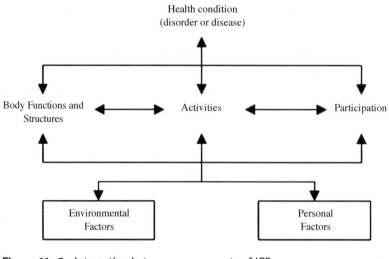

Figure 11–3. Interaction between components of ICF.

experience, medical condition, social environment), in order to find *directions* to improve, rehabilitate, sustain, or mediate *present or future functioning*. Understanding the *background and present functioning* is therefore an important part of what an AAC evaluation is about. This brings us to the discussion of whether there are *prerequisites* for AAC. Strictly speaking, the existence of prerequisites would mean that a person needs to meet certain criteria *before* AAC can even be considered. This has been called the *candidacy model* within AAC (Hourcade, Everhart Pilotte, West, & Parette, 2004). Do we expect an individual to present specific minimum levels of functioning in order to make AAC intervention doable and worthwhile? The answer is no! There are no strict prerequisites for the introduction of AAC. Here are the reasons why. In the *first* place, AAC includes techniques and intervention strategies that are specifically geared at the needs of individuals who function at the earliest developmental levels of communication (i.e., the nonintentional

prelinguistic level [see chapter 6]). *Second*, the very essence of AAC is that it is meant to help individuals for whom traditional methods won't provide sufficient help. In some cases, AAC may be nothing more or less than the last-resort help. Denying this help would be a transgression of the ethical principle that human communication is a right and assistance must be provided. *Third*, human communication is an essential part of what it means to be human. Communication plays a crucial role in what you are and what person (with knowledge and skills) you become. Helping to establish and improve human communication is, therefore, an act of recognition of human dignity. *Finally*, the reason why AAC should never be withheld from individuals relates to the fact that in typical development, communication is one of the driving forces, not just a result of other underlying components. In an excellent article titled, "Early Cognitive Skills as Prerequisites to Augmentative and Alternative Communication Use: What Are We Waiting For?," Kangas and Lloyd (1988) explain that interaction/communication and cognition are in a mutual developmental relationship. Cognition fires up communication, and vice versa. Therefore, it is not only ethically wrong to deny AAC to a person who is in the earliest stages of development, it also would reflect a misunderstanding of developmental dynamics.

3. Communicative Behavior Is Measurable

This principle may appear the most trivial but, at the same time, it is very essential. In interactions with parents and caregivers, one often comes across opinions that reflect a rather vague concept of how communication as a concept translates into behavior. When a well-intentioned teacher observes that "this student has little communication," it is often helpful to engage in a discussion introducing questions like, "What exactly is it that this student fails to communicate?" or "How often do you experience that you don't get your point across to this student?" Such questions can be attempts to move to an *operationalization* and a *quantification* of communication.

Operationalization

Operationalization is a term used in theoretical methodology to refer to the process of converting a concept into something "you can operate upon." In general, you try to make a concept concrete. Most of the time, you want to break the concept down into components that are measurable and quantifiable.

The big question is, of course, what the components of communication are. Here are a number of possible candidate components, all of which have been suggested in the literature on communication development: (1) intentionality, (2) number of words a person knows, (2) the degree of socialization a person has, (4) syntactic skills, and (5) pragmatic skills.

A few comments are needed here. When reviewing these candidate components, one needs to introduce the notions of *necessary* and *sufficient* components. From our earlier discussion of prelinguistic communication, we already know that word knowledge (or any other specific linguistic skill) is not considered to be a necessary condition for communication. When assessing communication, it is important to distinguish between these necessary components and others. Second, each of these (or other) components will need to be operationalized too, and are analyzed or broken down into subcomponents. Operationalization leads to a *construct*. A *construct* is a theoretical framework of measurable components. When you conduct an assessment, you—often implicitly—work from a construct.

Quantification

An important element that goes with measurability is quantification. This makes it possible to compare behaviors. In traditional psychometrics, test psychologists often work with *norms* and *normative tests* that compare a person's performance on a task with the performance of an age group, or another comparison or control group. This approach is valuable as it helps to appraise a person's behavior in a developmental or functional framework. Interpretation of such data is easier if the person's functional condition is similar to those of the comparison sample group. For example, if you compare a nondisabled middle class youngster with the sample group, you have a good chance to obtain a fair view of the person's skills and potential. However, as soon as you have a person whose developmental or functional condition is less comparable with the sample group (let's take a person with a disability—or a person from a linguistic, ethnical, or cultural minority), all kinds of caveats are needed when you want to interpret the results of the test. This is certainly the case for most (if not all) of the individuals who require an AAC evaluation. It is most likely that nearly each one of them presents with a unique combination of linguistic, socialization, perceptual, cognitive, and physical background idiosyncrasies, and therefore that the use of norm-referenced tests will only have a limited value. This is not to say that these tests should not be used (on the contrary); it mainly tells us to be careful with the interpretation of the results.

Can We Predict the Future?

While an AAC evaluation needs to look at the past to understand the present, the main focus is the future. We want to know if a person can be helped with AAC in general, and specifically what kind of AAC intervention (manual signs, a speech generating device, graphic symbols, etc.) has a good chance to help the person. How do our observations of the assessment of clients (the performance on the tasks we present them with) relate to potential future behavior of these clients as AAC users? That is the question of the validity of our assessment. We can distinguish between different types of validity. First, there is *face validity*. We obtain face validity if there is an obvious, almost intuitively understandable relation between the tasks and the projected future behavior. Presenting the clients with a

device and asking them to use it during the assessment session clearly has strong face validity. In this case, we are asking the client to do exactly what we anticipate will need to be done once a device would be prescribed for the client. However, as often in life, what is intuitively clear may be deceiving. If we present a communication device to a person for the very first time, how can we expect that a person will display the skills that normally will only develop after a period of learning and familiarization with the device?

On the other hand, other behaviors that have less intuitive face validity could be stronger predictors. Take for example, a memory test. If you ask a person to remember under which pile you have placed a card with a picture (face down) of a train, and under which pile you have placed a card with a picture of a spoon (again face down), it looks like you are testing the person's skills in a good old memory game, rather than testing AAC skills. However, in order to navigate through the pages of some of the communication devices, the user will need to remember where the messages are stored—which resembles the skills needed to play the good old memory game! However, not everyone believes this. Some AAC experts assume that a skilled device user relies on something that is more similar to motor learning. Nondisabled experienced computer keyboard users can have a typing speed of more than 100 words a minute, but may be unable to tell you where the letter "h" is on the keyboard if you would ask them. The location of the letters is stored in motor memory, and is less available to conscious reflection (at least less fast). If something similar occurs in AAC device use, we need to be careful in predicting a person's navigation skills based on semantic location memory. Note that this concept is one of the underlying principles of the motor planning approach in AAC device learning (Center for AAC and Autism, 2009).

This brings us to the concept of *predictive validity*. Unfortunately, at this point the literature does not provide us with a wealth of information regarding the predictive power of our assessments. The reason for this is probably very simple: communication relies on a configuration of many components (language, social skills, speed, intentionality, and personality traits). The success of AAC also depends on many factors outside of these communication components—which makes prediction hard. One of the saddest AAC realities is the high percentage of AAC abandonment; the fact that, despite laudable efforts by clinicians and others, clients and their communication partners are often not using and implementing the opportunities that were expected to come with AAC. Why is that? One suspected reason is that AAC abandonment often results from the subjective perception that the user (and their partners) does not receive a sufficient "return on investment." The costs of using AAC for the user can include: (1) learning new operational skills (learning manual signs, learning to operate the device), (2) learning new pragmatic skills (asking for patience, striking a good balance between eye contact with the partner, and looking at the communication device), (3) memorizing the location of prestored messages, (4) remembering the code of icon sequencing, and (5) using a device/method about which the person may have ambiguous feelings concerning social acceptability (does the device increase or decrease social stigmatization?).

Ironically, one of the costs for the AAC user may be the gain of independency. If people have experienced not being in charge for an extended period (because of the inability to communicate), they may feel intimidated by the expectation that they are now expected to make choices and answer questions.

The costs of introduction of AAC for the communication partners are somewhat similar; it can require them to learn new skills (e.g., learn manual signs, learn how to maintain a device—don't forget to charge the batteries at night!) and new attitudes (ask and wait—a long time—for a response). Things go by so much faster when you do not need to ask and you can just do what needs to be done. Communication is a process that is shared by sender and receiver. If things go slow for the sender, they automatically go slow for the receiver too. Just like the use of a device or manual signs may or may not be socially acceptable by the person with AAC needs, it may also be felt to be cumbersome by the communication partner.

Maybe the most important validity related concept here is *construct validity*. This is the term used to indicate how strong the relation is between the theoretical construct (communication) and its operationalizations (what does it mean to be a good communicator). In other words, if we define and decide what behaviors are the indicators of communication, our assessment will have validity if they measure exactly these behaviors.

The reason why AAC assessment is still somewhat of a vague process and concept is, without any doubt, the fact that there are no clear norms with which to compare the client's performance. However, the search for norms for AAC performance may remain forever unrealistic because: (1) communication is multifactorial (at most, one might seek to find norms for individual factors) and (2) each individual AAC candidate presents with a unique configuration of skills and abilities.

This makes it hard to evaluate or judge individual progress (and, indirectly, to set intervention goals). Take, for example, a 5-year-old girl who has learned and is using between 75 and 100 messages that have been programmed on her speech-generating communication device. Is this a high or low achiever? How many new words/messages should she be able to learn within the next year? At this point, we simply lack the norms (or even the conceptual framework) to answer this question in a sensible way.

4. AAC Is Partially Measurable Through the Assessment of Language Components such as Vocabulary

We fortunately have a number of highly valuable speech and language tests that can be used within AAC. However, one should be reminded of two important caveats: (1) the language acquisition conditions are likely to be incomparable to those of the typically speaking and language using population, and (2) the fact that most AAC candidates have limited access to natural speech necessitates caution when interpreting spoken language production.

(1) *The language acquisition conditions are likely to be incomparable to those of the normal speaking and language using population.* Standardized tests have been normed on typically developing and functioning population samples (i.e., children and adults who have been fully exposed to language and, most importantly, have had no limitations in the use of expressive spoken language). AAC candidates usually don't fit this developmental or functional profile—therefore, the use

of the norms should be used in a somewhat informative (but not explanatory) manner (i.e., it can inform you where the person's language production would be situated *if it were* a reflection of a typical development).

(2) *The fact that most AAC candidates have limited access to natural speech necessitates caution when interpreting spoken language production.* Even if an AAC user has found an alternative for natural speech (manual signs, a speech-generating device), it is unlikely that the experience of the alternative form of communication matches typical spoken language production. In general, AAC users speak less than typical speakers. A typical 6-year-old may "speak" thousands of words a day. A simple observation of the efforts and the opportunities of AAC users to talk (remember, AAC use often requires more effort; also there may not always be a patient audience for the AAC user) makes it clear that even in the best conditions, an AAC user's opportunities and expressive language practice will not come close to those of typical users (Proctor & Zangari, 2009).

DYNAMIC ASSESSMENT

Assessment of the needs for AAC of individuals with no functional speech is a difficult task for a number of reasons. Often, the person has not had much experience with any device or communication tool, which makes it hard to assess his or her potential for learning. For this reason, it is useful to have tools that allow the examiner to conduct dynamic assessment. Dynamic assessment is focused on the learning potential of the learner, rather than on the actual level of knowledge or skill. Dynamic assessment is a systematic way of predicting and measuring what a person can do. However, assessment is not or should not be some form of shooting in the dark. When trying out and measuring a person's potential (and, in the case of communication, the potential of the communication partners), the steps that are taken should be based on a view of: (1) the skills needed for the behavior, (2) factors contributing to the behavior (such as motivation and opportunity), (3) the person's individual strengths and weaknesses (both mentally and physically), and (4) the availability of communication solutions (funding, devices, knowledge). *Dynamic assessment* is an approach to the evaluation of a person's learning potential by teaching and presenting the person with a series of learning experiences and observing whether a person shows evidence of learnability. In many cases, an important portion of AAC assessment will be dynamic for two reasons. *First*, as one has to introduce new skills (e.g., imitating a gesture, operating a device), measurement can only follow introduction of teaching and learning. *Second*, as (especially nonverbal) communication is largely idiosyncratic (i.e., everyone has developed a personal style of expressing needs and opinions nonverbally), there is no comparability that is expressed in norms (Snell, 2002).

Bringing AAC devices into the assessment room and trying out how, on the spot, a client navigates the aid and succeeds in touching the screen and making the device generate words, is a straightforward example of dynamic approach. In a more systematic way, new communicative behaviors (a manual sign, the activation of a switch) is part of a process in which a clinician (and a team) gains insight in the communication learning potential of a cli-

ent. In children, such an approach can be play-based (Uys & Alant, 2004).

MEASURING INSTRUMENTS

Besides observation, dynamic assessment trials, and interviews, clinicians can use standardized or semistandardized instruments to help to obtain a profile of the AAC user or candidate.

Table 11–1 gives an overview and some examples of: (1) general development measurements, (2) tools to measure communication behavior, and (3) language performance tests.

MEASURING COMMUNICATION AS PART OF A DEVELOPMENTAL COMPONENT

It is important that the clinician appraises the developmental background and learning opportunities in order to understand communicative needs. Lack of communication limits developmental potential. Therefore, one should look at the possibility that communication may have been withheld from the person (sometimes well intended) due to misperception of the person's abilities, or to protective measures, or simply due to lack of experiences. The provision of AAC can accelerate development and unlock cognitive potential. For example, Goossens' (1989) reports on a 6-year-old nonspeaking girl with cerebral palsy, who was considered to be severally intellectually disabled. However, after 7 months of intensive intervention with eye-gaze training, switch use, and graphic symbol communication, the same girl was identified to have a normal intelligence.

Table 11–1. Classification of Assessment Tools and Examples

	General Development Instruments	Communication Behavior Instruments	Language Behavior Instruments
Non-AAC Specific	Bayley	CSBS	CELF
	Battelle	MacArther-Bates CDI	Peabody
			Fluharty
			Bankson
AAC-Specific		Communication Sampling and Analysis (CSA)	
		Communication Matrix	
		Communication Competence Profile	
		Triple-C Checklist	
		TASP (Bruno)	
		Snell-Loncke	
		AAC Profile: Continuum of Learning	

Throughout life, communication and cognition go hand-in-hand. Cognition feeds communication (our understanding makes us ask questions and make comments about the world), and communication is the fuel for cognition. This is never more the case than in the earliest developmental stages. When assessing a person's need, it is essential to understand a person's cognitive level and intelligence. Psychological assessment of developmental level and components can include tests (e.g., the Bayley Scales of Infant Development, the Vineland Adaptive Behavior Scales, and the Wechsler Intelligence Scale for Children (WISC-R/revised version).

COMMUNICATION COMPETENCE PROFILE

Hans van Balkom and the Dutch AAC team around Radboud University in Nijmegen (the Netherlands; e.g., Stoep, Deckers, Van Zaalen, Van Balkom, & Verhoeven, 2012) have developed a measurement tool that tries to grasp the different components of communication in a "Communication Competence Profile" (CCP; Figure 11–4). It operationalizes the principle that communicative competence must be a multidimensional construct to which different subskills (linguistic, cognitive, social, perceptual) contribute. The instrument records information in a number of domains. The domains are perception, memory, cognition, sensorimotor level, language comprehension and production, vocabulary, morphosyntax, communication, and socialemotional functioning. The scores of the different sections provide a profile that help teams to decide on the content and the priorities for an intervention plan.

The profile allows inspection of strengths and potential threats to growth (SWOT: Strengths, Weaknesses, Opportunities, and Threats). The system also

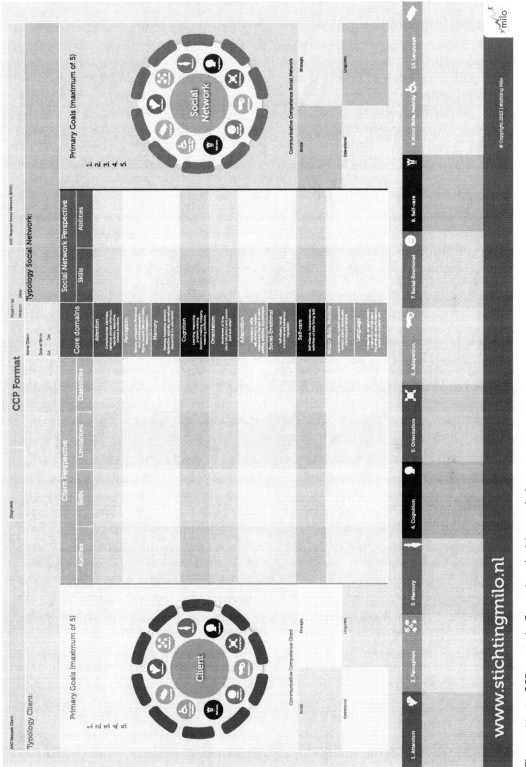

Figure 11–4. CCP example. Reproduced with permission.

encourages the formulation of SMART (Specific, Measurable, Acceptable, Realistic, and Time; O'Neill, Conzemius, Commodore, & Pulsfus, 2006) goals. CCP is obviously a powerful instrument for measurement as a dynamic continuously adjusting process performed jointly by the client, the client's communication partners, and the surrounding team. Such instruments certainly have the potential of a framework that will help build data, that will allow data mining, which in turn will help to determine construct validity (e.g., which components within the concept of communication competence weigh more, etc.).

ASSESSMENT OF PRELINGUISTIC AND EARLY LINGUISTIC FUNCTIONING

As explained in Chapter 6, a range of AAC techniques can be used to help individuals who function at an early stage of communication. Most of the times, intervention and measurement/assessment will be intertwined. To gather detailed information of individuals functioning at the *prelinguistic or early linguistic level*, the following (nonexhaustive list of) tests can be useful:

Communication and Symbolic Behavior Scales (Wetherby & Prizant, 2002): This standardized instrument is increasingly used to assess young children who are considered at risk for language and communicative development.

MacArthur-Bates Communicative Development Inventories (Fenson et al., 2007): These standardized inventories consist of a "words and gestures form" (for the typical population between 8 and 18 months) and a "words and sentences form" (for the typical population between 16 and 30 months).

The *Snell-Loncke questionnaire* is a nonstandardized exploratory instrument to be used within the framework of dynamic assessment of children at the presymbolic and early symbolic level (Snell & Loncke, 2005, see http://people.virginia.edu/~mes5l/manual9-02.pdf).

The *Inventory of Potential Communicative Acts* (IPCA) is a questionnaire developed by Sigafoos, Arthur-Kelly, and Butterfield (2006) to analyze behavior that has communicative potential. The instrument helps caregivers to identify behaviors that can be modulated and shaped into acceptable and effective communication.

The *Communication Matrix* is an online instrument developed by Charity Rowland (http://www.communication-matrix.org) that generates a profile of the first stages of communicative (presymbolic and early symbolic) development. The profile can be used for intervention planning and for keeping track of progress and development (Rowland, 2011; Rowland & Fried-Oken, 2010).

Communication Sampling and Analysis is a tool developed by Marilyn Buzolich and her team. It samples observable interaction between the person and the partner. The focus is on the interaction itself, not just the behavior of the person. The means of interaction are described, as well as their functionality (how well they work). This sampling is used to generate intervention options to extend the scope of interaction (means and effects; Buzolich, 2011; see http://csa.acts-at.com/csa-info.html).

The *Test for Early Communication and Emerging Language* (TECEL) can be administered from infancy to the age of 48 months. It is one of the few tests especially developed to assess receptive and expressive skills of nonspeaking children.

An earlier version of the TECEL used to be known as the *Nonspeech Test for Receptive and Expressive Language* by Mary Blake Huer, published first in 1983 (Huer, 1983; Huer & Miller, 2011).

The *Triple C—Checklist of Communicative Competencies* (Iacono, West, Bloomberg, & Johnson, 2009) is an Australian instrument that allows to determine levels and sublevels of unintentional communication in individuals of all ages with severe intellectual disabilities.

LANGUAGE TESTS AND THEIR USABILITY

General language tests can be useful within AAC assessment, although caution needs to be a guiding factor when interpreting the results. There is no general "best choice" or "fit for all." Some of the better known tests include:

The *Peabody Picture Vocabulary Test* is an attempt to measure receptive vocabulary. The test is sometimes used to measure verbal intelligence, especially in individuals with limited expressive skills. It has a strong focus on word recognition. Other important language functions (syntactical-combinatorial skills, for example) are not in the focus.

The *Preschool Language Scale* attempts to measure a more comprehensive configuration of language components. It is aimed at children in the preschool developmental stage. The authors present the data and the scores in a milestone-oriented framework.

Other useful language tests include the *Fluharty Preschool Speech and Language Screening Test*, the *Bankson Language Screening Test*, and the *Batelle Developmental Inventory Screening Test*. The clinician—often in consultation with other professionals —will determine which tests are most likely to provide critical information.

Are standardized and norm-referenced language tests appropriate for AAC evaluations? They can certainly be used as clinical-diagnostic tools to gain insight in linguistic and potential communication, but one needs to be careful with the interpretation of the results (Downing, 2009). Norm-referenced instruments intend to provide a comparison with typically developing peers (i.e., individuals who do not have communication limitations and have learned and developed skills through daily interaction with their environment). The condition of the typical AAC user does not allow comparison. With all the caveats concerning their direct applicability toward individuals with AAC needs, these and other language development tests can nevertheless provide the AAC clinician with important information about level of functioning.

MEASURING OF SPECIFIC AAC RELATED SKILLS

The use and success of AAC rely on several skills. Although our body of knowledge is still very limited, research studies and clinical (and educational) experiences have identified a number of skills that may be critical for the use of communication devices. These skills include (but are not limited to) symbol awareness, choice making, short-term visual and auditory memory, and combinatorial capacity (to form sentences). Some instruments have been developed with a special focus on identifying the needs and specific skills for AAC users. In collaboration with Mayer-Johnson, LLC, Joan Bruno developed the

Test of Aided-Communication Symbol Performance. This test uses graphic symbols and communication boards in a step-by-step format. The purpose is to determine a child's potential to learn and use graphic symbols in communication. The test consists of four subtests: (1) symbol size and number, (2) grammatical encoding, (3) categorization, and (4) syntactic performance (Bruno & Trembath, 2006).

At the University of Virginia, Loncke and colleagues works with clinicians from 10 different countries to develop a *Graphic symbol assessment tool.* This tool was constructed through a series of expert evaluations of four consecutive versions of the instrument. In its 2014 edition, the test consists of the following subtests: symbol identification, symbol preference, symbol memory, functional recognition, classification and association, phrase repetition with graphic symbols, symbol combination, and literacy (Loncke, Davis, & Poppalardo, 2011).

At the Centre for Augmentative and Alternative Communication in Pretoria (South Africa), Uys and colleagues (in press) developed the *Pretoria Test for AAC,* a test that is geared toward specific AAC skills in school-age children.

Augmentative and Alternative Communication Profile. A Continuum of Learning (Kovach, 2009) is an instrument to measure development and progress in the four areas of communicative competence as proposed by Light (1989; linguistic, operational, strategic, and social competence). The scale identifies five developmental steps within each type of competence.

Social Networks: A Communication Inventory for Individuals with Complex Communication Needs and Their Communication Partners. This questionnaire allows to obtain an overview of the differential styles and use of communication means by the person and his or her communication partners depending on the familiarity and characteristics of situations and partners (see also Chapter 12; Blackstone & Hunt-Berg, 2003).

CONDUCTING AN EVALUATION

How do we plan an AAC evaluation? Much will depend on background information which is available. Here is a list of components that will help you decide what will be the likely components of your evaluation.

1. *Information gathering.* Interview and observation of the client, the parents, and/or the spouse. What has triggered the interest in an AAC evaluation? Have there been previous AAC evaluations and AAC interventions? If so, did they lead to improvement and satisfaction? If information can be disclosed, information about linguistic, communicative, cognitive, social, and relational functioning is important. If the client is a child, educational and academic data may be helpful. If an adult, information of onset and course of condition, as well as professional and rehabilitation progress is helpful.
2. *Also, we need to make sure that everything is clear regarding who will pay for the evaluation* (insurance policies, school, Medicare/ Medicaid).
3. *The person's preferences, interests, and needs.* This information can be gathered through interview and observation. It can also help in assessing motivation, including the willingness to learn new ways to communicate.
4. *Hearing and vision status.* The evaluation needs not only to measure sound

reception but also auditory speech perception. Indications about progressive hearing or vision loss are extremely important.

5. *Physical abilities and mobility.* This information is needed in case AAC solutions will be needed that require adapted forms of physical access. Assessment of physical possibilities will help to determine which physical access alternatives should be pursued. Data on body posture, body orientation, seating, and positioning will play a role in determining the assessment.

6. *Cognitive and developmental level.* When performing an AAC evaluation, one needs to know if a person has reached a level of sustained attention, understanding of intentionality, symbolic awareness, word knowledge, and memory skills (this is important for navigation requirements).

7. *Linguistic level.* AAC candidates have, almost by definition, an extremely limited expressive language. However the discrepancy between expressive and receptive language can be considerable. The assessment will need to explore the person's receptive knowledge and understanding of words, messages, and syntactic structures.

8. *Reading assessment* (Koppenhaver, Foley, & Williams, 2009). For obvious reasons, the literacy level and skills of a person can make a difference in determining which AAC solutions are the most appropriate and functional for a person.

9. *Nonverbal and nontech spontaneous communication.* Reported use of gestures, pointing, and drawing as improvised forms of augmentative communication can be interpreted as indications of AAC learning potential.

10. *Experience with augmentative communication and devices.* During the assessment, one can observe the client with a range of communication devices. Insurance agencies will require that you try out several nontech and low-tech solutions and evaluate if and motivate why these are not preferred over a more complex device.

   Besides this requirement of motivation by the funding agencies, this is a difficult part of the assessment. In many cases, you want to determine the clients' potential to familiarize themselves with complex devices that not only implies the development of a whole new set of operational competencies, but also a shift in communication pragmatics (taking on a more assertive and active role in communication). The predictive validity of any assessment of a totally new configuration of skills is always limited.

11. *An assessment of present and future needs and potential.* AAC evaluation should not (only) be about the present, but (also) about the future. AAC aims at liberating the person from (some of) the limitations of communication. Often, the clients and their communication partners have already been able to develop daily strategies to get by for most daily routines (getting up in the morning, meals, TV, etc.), but they could have given up on talks about more complex (and more interesting) matters, or they may have stopped inviting friends over (or expecting that the person with AAC needs will actually be part of the conversation). In other words, AAC assessment must be about the vision of what we think is doable, what is reachable. Of course, this should not be just wishful thinking or dreaming, but it should be

part of a realistic assessment of a person's learnability.

12. *The resourcefulness and motivation of the person's environment to learn together with the client and to engage in new forms and ways of interaction.* This is sometimes a challenge. For example, if a client is a resident of a nursing home, the opportunities of interaction with caregivers may be limited (due to staff work schedules) unless the person can rely on pleasant conversations with other residents, visiting relatives and friends, or other volunteer visitors.

FUNCTIONAL, DEVELOPMENTAL, AND DYNAMIC INTERPRETATION OF THE DATA

Zabala (2005) has developed "SETT" as a framework to plan assessment of special needs (including AAC needs) from a dynamic functional and developmental perspective. SETT stands for "Student —Environment—Task—Tools." This framework is a great reminder of the fact that functional communication (and the prediction of what will be needed in the future, and the prediction of its success) is dependent on several factors. The *student* (for our terminology: the *client*; Sett) presents with specific characteristics that needs to be assessed. They include the person's learning ability, preferences and interests, physical abilities (and physical access!), language level, expressive forms of language, and actual forms of communication (Table 11–2). For the latter, the following overview of forms may be useful (Table 11–3). The *environment* (sEtt) includes an assessment of places, physical arrangements, (in)dependence on technology, and supporting strategies by the communication partners. Under physical arrangements, special attention is needed for seating and positioning. Occupational therapists can be supportive in helping to find seating and physical positioning that allows a person to assume a comfortable, physical (eye-to-eye, if possible), interactive position with the environment, with comfortable and unstressed muscle tone.

Table 11–2. Overview of Preferences

Please check all that apply	Close Family Members (parents)	Good Friends and Relatives	Acquaintances (classmates)	Paid Workers (teacher, attendant)	Unfamiliar People (store clerks)
Eye gaze					
Facial expressions/body language					
Gestures					
Pointing to objects, places					
Pointing to photos, pictures					
Vocalizations (i.e., speech sounds not always understood by others)					
Manual sign language/sign language approximations					

Table 11–2. *continued*

Verbal speech—single words					
Verbal speech—two words together					
Verbal speech—three words or more together					
Word approximations					
Writing/drawing					
Communication board/book with photos					
Communication board/book with pictures					
Communication board/book with words and alphabet (reading, spelling)					
Simple communication device—**describe**:					
Complex communication device—**describe**:					
Special communication software used on a computer— **Name of software:**					
Phone					
E-mail					
Combination of methods—**describe**:					
Other—**describe**:					

What methods and tools has the child *tried* in the past but is *no longer* using:

Please rate how well the child's communication is understood:

1	2	3	4	5

Source: From Children's Treatment Network of Simcoe York (Canada): AAC Guided Assessment (Daily Communication Partners, September 2007).

Table 11–3. Tool Selection Table for the SETT Framework

Type of Tool	For Input (Partner uses to help child understand)	For Output (Child uses to help partner understand)
No-Tech Strategies: (i.e., gestures, eye gaze, facial expressions, body language, partner strategies, sign language, etc.)		
Low-Tech Tools: (i.e., visual supports, schedules, communication board/book, picture exchange, etc.)		
High-Tech Tools: (i.e., speech-generating devices, computer equipment, switches, special mouse, etc.)		

Source: Reprinted with permission http://www.joyzabala.com

Tasks are the routines and the activities that people engage in—or the activities that they *wish* to engage in. We need to remember that one of our goals with AAC is to broaden the person's range of action and possibilities. Therefore, in our assessment, we should not only look at what the people are able to do now, but also what they would like to be able to do. The challenge of AAC intervention will be to remove barriers so that the person will be able to do more. Finally, under *tools*, we need to list: (1) what the person is presently using, and (2) what we recommend that the person and his or her environment and communication partners *learn* to use (see Table 11–3).

Feature Matching

How to avoid losing yourself in the forest of AAC solutions, AAC devices, and AAC technology? The best approach may be the feature-approach, where one simply makes a list of all the characteristics of a device—which will help to decide and motivate a choice one makes for a client. In AAC, this "feature matching" approach has often been advocated. Lloyd, Fuller, and Arvidson (1997) define feature matching as "a process in which an AAC user's current and projected needs are matched to features of AAC symbols and devices." Because no AAC symbol set/system or device may have all of the desired features, selections that have the most desirable features for an AAC user's needs are made to achieve "goodness of fit" (Lloyd et al., 1997, p. 530).

In other words, this approach seeks to identify the cognitive, linguistic, and social strengths and weaknesses of the person together with the motor-operational skills, and link these with the motor, cognitive and other requirements of an AAC system or method. If a person shows to have a good understanding of graphic representations, graphic symbols may be a good choice to be used in communication.

However, although this approach makes decisions workable and easier to motivate (and is probably the best possible), one needs to remember that a device (nor its user) should not be considered as just the sum of its characteristics. Whether a person will be able to successfully operate an AAC device cannot be entirely predicted until the person has been using the device for a while. For example, take memory: it is clear that memory is needed when you have to navigate through your device to the right page. But how can we know that someone will have a good "AAC display memory"? It would be naïve to suppose that any general memory test would be able to do this very specific job.

MULTIDISCIPLINARY

As for the logistics of the assessment, an AAC evaluation will, in most cases, need to take a multidisciplinary approach. The number one person in the team is the client. Throughout the evaluation, the professionals will try to solicit the clients' opinion about what they think will work, what they like, and what they don't like, or what they are missing. Throughout the AAC evaluation, it is a good custom to provide explanations of what you intend to do ("Now I am going to see if you can use this device. You can make this device speak for you. Let's try," and "I would like to see if you can remember which pile I placed these plates with pictures. A memory game, you see. When you use a device, you also need to remember where the pictures are stored"). Often, the client may not be able to process all the information that you are providing. This is one of the reasons why, in general, it is good to conduct the evaluation in the presence of a parent, a spouse, a relative, and

sometimes a teacher or another speech-language pathologist. These communication partners are not there just to observe, but to participate. Their involvement in the assessment generally helps you to identify cooperative strategies between partner and client. Besides the client's communicative partners, assessment should often include professionals from other disciplines: occupational therapist, physical therapist, early intervention specialist, or teacher. Occasionally you can have other professionals involved (e.g., nurse or reading specialist).

INTERESTED PARTIES

There are a few words to be said about the involvement of vendors or representatives of manufacturers of communication devices. While it is good to know the representatives of the main companies that serve your region, when it comes to providing services (including an AAC evaluation), it is imperative that the relationship is professional and ethically correct. Often representatives have such extensive experience with service provision—they may have seen and read hundreds of reports—that it is tempting to solicit their help and presence during an AAC evaluation. It should not be forgotten that the AAC evaluation must bear all the professional integrity of the speech-language pathologist and the team. Many funding agencies require an explicit statement from the speech-language pathologist stating that there is not a conflict of interest between your assessment and your choices for recommendation and prescriptions. With that in mind, it should be said that a professional relationship with the representatives of device manufacturers is highly recommendable. For example, they can help the professional clinician with finding ways to obtain a loan device. As said, very often it is impossible to know how well a device "fits" a person unless you can allow the person and his or her communication partners to use and explore the device during some time. The manufacturing companies often will also provide help with the process of submitting documents for Medicare (or other insurance) approval for a device. Often their websites will show you models of reports of AAC evaluations.

New Ways of Assessment and Data Gathering

Major changes are taking place in the practice of client-related data gathering and data management. Client-related data can be stored in central electronic databases. Increasingly, health administrators, educators, and clinicians are moving toward using online data collecting as intervention decisions are made, while entering and interpreting new data coming in with each clinical intervention and assessment session.

This practice is already blooming in the field of diagnostic (neuro-) psychological assessment (Pearson, 2013). This brings along challenges and possibilities. The challenge is related to the risks of insufficient safeguarding of private and confidential information of clients (Houston, Stredler-Brown, & Alverson, 2012).

The advantages are at least twofold. First, it allows forms of telepracticing in which the person with the expertise (e.g., suggestions about which decisions to make for AAC solutions) can be at a distance from the client. Second, it makes it possible to contribute to larger databases, which can be critical to: (1) discern patterns of communication behaviors and profiles (which are typically considered to be unique and idiosyncratic), and (2) better predict outcomes based on more extensive evidence. As mentioned before, this is the approach taken by new projects such as the *Communication Matrix* (see http://www.communicationmatrix.org).

For years, technology has allowed device users to record their ongoing expressive production into a communication log, which could be analyzed and used for intervention decisions at any point (e.g., Language Activity Monitor/Data logging) by retrieving the data from the device. At present, these same functions and measurements are possible through cloud computing (Gomory & Steele, 2012; see also Figure 3–5 in Chapter 3).

Centralized databases may be a solution for one of the biggest problems of AAC: the uniqueness and lack of comparability of one's client's results.

Costs and Funding

What is the cost of AAC and who pays for it? Depending on the individual case, AAC can be seen as an aid to foster development (e.g., in young children), as an education tool (in school children), or as a rehabilitation measure. Regardless of these different perspectives and situations, AAC is much more than a method or a device. AAC service delivery is a process in which users work together with their natural communication partners (parents, relatives, friends, colleagues), under the advice from an expert or expert team. The responsibility and the intensity of team-guided intervention can vary enormously. There are many cases where it is perfectly responsible, and the right thing to do to simply hand over the device to a user, who will independently decide when, where, and how to use the device. On the other hand, there are also many cases where AAC introduction requires coaching, technical instructions, and modeling. Introduction of AAC and devices is part of a clinical, an educational, or a rehabilitation intervention program. Depending on documented necessities and regulations, governmental institutions, insurance companies, or educational agencies (e.g., school districts) can fund expenses for AAC assessment and for purchase of dedicated AAC devices (Golinker, 2009).

POINTS TO REMEMBER

- The purpose of assessment in AAC is to determine *if* a person can benefit from AAC, *what* AAC intervention should consist of, and what the *predictions* for functioning with AAC would be.
- "Communication skills" is a theoretical construct that can be described as a set of mental and human abilities, which can be analyzed and measured as separate components.
- The following components need to be addressed in assessments of a person's potential use of AAC: cognitive operations, linguistic operations, motor operations, perceptual operations, and social-pragmatic operations.
- Light (1989) has proposed to break communicative competence into linguistic competence, operational competence, social competence, and strategic competence.
- Assessment of present behavior and skills needs to be interpreted in terms of functionality. Observation of today's behavior and skills will provide information on the possibilities to acquire new behaviors and new skills.
- Communicative behavior is measurable.
- AAC is partially measurable through the assessment of language components.
- Dynamic assessment is the term used to indicate an approach to evaluate a person's learning potential by teaching and presenting the person with a series of learning experiences and observing whether a person shows evidence of learnability.
- General language tests can be useful within AAC assessment as long as one takes into account that the AAC user presents with a likely different profile than the people on whom the test has been normed.
- Feature matching is a process in which an AAC user's current and projected needs are matched to features of AAC symbols and devices.

REFERENCES

Blackstone, S., & Hunt-Berg, M. (2003). *Social networks: A communication inventory for individuals with complex communication needs and their communication partners manual.* Monterey, CA: Augmentative Communication.

Bruno, J., & Trembath, D. (2006). Use of aided language stimulation to improve syntactic performance during a weeklong intervention program. *AAC: Augmentative and Alternative Communication, 22*(4), 300–313.

Buzolich, M. J. (2011). *CSA: Communication sampling and analysis.* San Francisco, CA: Augmentative Communication and Technology Services.

Center for AAC and Autism. (2009). *What is LAMP? (language acquisition through motor planning).* Retrieved from http://www.aacandautism.com/lamp

Downing, J. (2009). Assessment of early communication skills. In G. Soto & C. Zangari (Eds.), *Practically speaking. Language, literacy, and academic development for students with AAC needs* (pp. 27–46). Baltimore, MD: Paul H. Brookes.

Fenson, L., Marchman, V. A., Thal, D., Dale, P., Reznick, J., & Bates, E. (2007). *The MacArthur-Bates Communicative Development Inventories: User's guide and technical manual* (2nd ed.). Baltimore, MD: Paul H. Brookes.

Frith, C., & Frith, U. (2005). Theory of mind. *Current Biology, 15*(17), R644–R645.

Golinker, L. (2009). Speech generating device funding for children. *Exceptional Parent, 39*(9), 64–65.

Gomory, A., & Steele, R. (2012). *Measurement, assessment, and data use cycles in electronically delivered aphasia rehabilitation offerings.* Presentation at the ISAAC Research Symposium, University of Pittsburgh, PA.

Goossens', C. (1989). Aided communication intervention before assessment: A case study of a child with cerebral palsy. *Augmentative and Alternative Communication, 5*(1), 14.

Hourcade, J., Everhart Pilotte, T., West, E., & Parette, P. (2004). A history of augmentative and alternative communication for individuals with severe and profound disabilities. *Focus on Autism and Other Developmental Disabilities, 19*(4), 235–244.

Houston, K. T., Stredler-Brown, A., & Alverson, D. C. (2012). More than 150 years in the making: The evolution of telepractice for hearing, speech, and language services. *Volta Review, 112*(3), 195–205.

Huer, M. (1983). *The Nonspeech Test for Receptive and Expressive Language.* Lake Zurich, IL: Don Johnston Developmental Equipment.

Huer, M., & Miller, L. (2011). *Test of Early Communication and Emerging Language (TECEL).* Austin, TX: Pro-Ed.

Iacono, T., West, D., Bloomberg, K., & Johnson, H. (2009). Reliability and validity of the revised triple C: Checklist of communicative competencies for adults with severe and multiple disabilities. *Journal of Intellectual Disability Research, 53*(1), 44–53.

Kangas, K. A., & Lloyd, L. L. (1988). Early cognitive skills as prerequisites to augmentative and alternative communication use: What are we waiting for? *Augmentative and Alternative Communication, 4*(4), 211.

Koppenhaver, D., Foley, B., & Williams, A. (2009). Diagnostic reading assessment for students with AAC needs. In G. Soto & C. Zangari (Eds.), *Practically speaking: Language, literacy, and academic development for students with AAC needs* (pp. 71–91). Baltimore, MD: Paul H. Brookes.

Kovach, T. (2009). *Augmentative and alternative communication profile: A continuum of learning.* East Moline, IL: LinguiSystems.

Light, J. (1989). Toward a definition of communicative competence for individuals using augmentative and alternative communication systems. *Augmentative and Alternative Communication, 5*(2), 137–144.

Lloyd, L., Fuller, D., & Arvidson, H. (Eds.). (1997). *Augmentative and alternative communication. A handbook of principles and practices.* Boston, MA: Allyn & Bacon.

Loncke, F., Davis, B., & Poppalardo, L. (2011). *The development of communication boards as assessment tools for AAC.* Presentation at the Annual Conference of the Speech-Language and Hearing Association of Virginia, Richmond, VA.

Murphy, J., & Boa, S. (2012). Using the WHO-ICF with talking mats to enable adults with long-term communication difficulties to participate in goal setting. *AAC: Augmentative and Alternative Communication, 28*(1), 52–60.

O'Neill, J., Conzemius, A., Commodore, C., & Pulsfus, C. (2006). *The power of SMART goals: Using goals to improve student learning.* Bloomington, IN: Solution Tree.

Pearson. (2013). *Online assessment.* Retrieved from http://downloads.pearsonassessments.com/videos/nextgeneration/NextGen_Roadmap/NextGen%20RoadmApp_web

Proctor, L., & Zangari, C. (2009). Language assessment for students who use AAC. In G. Soto & C. Zangari (Eds.), *Practically speaking. Language, literacy, and academic development for students with AAC needs* (pp. 47–69). Baltimore, MD: Paul H. Brookes.

Rosenbaum, P., & Stewart, D. (2004). The World Health Organization International Classification of Functioning, Disability, and Health: A model to guide clinical thinking, practice and research in the field of cerebral palsy. *Seminars in Pediatric Neurology. Current Perspectives in Cerebral Palsy, 11*(1), 5–10.

Rowland, C. (2011). Using the communication matrix to assess expressive skills in early communicators. *Communication Disorders Quarterly, 32*(3), 190–201.

Rowland, C. *Online communication matrix* [website]. Portland, OR: Oregon Health & Science University. Retrieved from http://communicationMatrix.org

Rowland, C., & Fried-Oken, M. (2010). Communication matrix: A clinical and research assessment tool targeting children with severe communication disorders. *Journal of Pediatric Rehabilitation Medicine, 3*(4), 319–329.

Rowland, C., Fried-Oken, M., Steiner, S., Lollar, D., Phelps, R., Simeonsson, R., & Granlund, M. (2012). Developing the ICF-CY for AAC profile and code set for children who rely on AAC. *AAC: Augmentative and Alternative Communication, 28*(1), 21–32.

Sigafoos, J., Arthur-Kelly, M., & Butterfield, N. (2006). Inventory of potential communicative acts (IPCA). In *Enhancing everyday communication* (pp. 137–153). Baltimore, MD: Paul H. Brookes.

Sigafoos, J., Woodyatt, G., Keen, D., Tait, K., Tucker, M., Roberts-Pennell, D., & Pittendreigh, N. (2000). Identifying potential communicative acts in children with developmental and physical disabilities. *Communication Disorders Quarterly, 21*(2), 77–86.

Snell, M. E. (2002). Using dynamic assessment with learners who communicate nonsymbolically. *AAC: Augmentative and Alternative Communication, 18*(3), 163–176.

Snell, M., & Loncke, F. (2005). *Manual for the dynamic assessment of nonsymbolic communication* (unpublished manuscript). [Translated into Spanish (March 2006) by the Department of Participation and Solidarity in Education in Andalucia, Motril/Granada, Spain.] http://people.virginia.edu/~mes51/manual9-02.pdf.

Sperber, D., & Wilson, D. (1986). *Relevance: Communication and cognition.* Oxford, UK: Blackwell.

Stoep, J., Deckers, S., Van Zaalen, Y., Van Balkom, H., & Verhoeven, L. (2012). *Profiling communicative competence: A neuro-socio-cognitive reasoning model for AAC assessment* (unpublished manuscript). Lecture presented at the Biennial Conference of the International Society for Augmentative and Alternative Communication, Pittsburgh, PA.

Uys, K., & Alant, E. (2004). Play-based assessment of communication-related skills in young children with disabilities: The validation of an assessment tool. *Perspectives in Education, 22*(2), 115–128.

Uys, C., Bornman, J., Samuels, A., Ledwaba, G., Hardy, M., & Tonsing, K. (in press). Assessment instrument: Augmentative and alternative communication system for the school context. In E. Moolman & J. Rose (Eds.), *AAC resource manual.* Pretoria, SA: Centre of AAC, University of Pretoria.

Wetherby, A. M., & Prizant, B. M. (2002). *Communication and symbolic behavior scales: Developmental profile* (1st normed ed.). Baltimore, MD: Paul H Brookes.

Zabala, J. S. (2005). *Using the SETT framework to level the learning field for students with disabilities* (unpublished manuscript).

CHAPTER 12

AAC and the Community

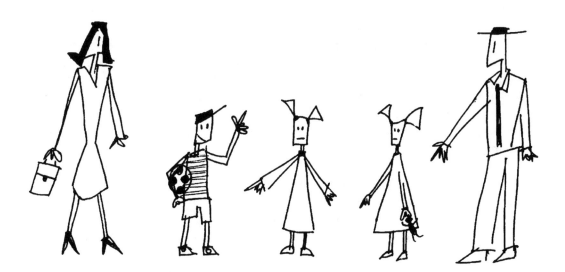

AAC is meant to provide a voice to individuals with no or limited speech skills. That is important because people want to be able to exert control over their environment. Indicating your needs, telling someone that you have enough, giving your two cents worth of opinion on something, telling someone you love them, are all ways of controlling our environment. We want people to do something, to stop doing it, or we want them to know something (often about us), and occasionally we try to influence how they think about

us or about anything. We use communication also to extract information by asking questions. Often we receive information without asking for it. All of that can be facilitated by AAC.

But why do we want that? Because we want to participate (i.e., we want to take part in the community). We want to have rich and enduring relationships with others. Social psychologists tell us that our desire to be part of the community goes back to a desire to be protected and safe. The ultimate test of the success of

AAC will, therefore, lie in the question of whether or not it does help individuals to participate in their communities.

To what degree and how well does AAC facilitate participation in the community? What research can help us to improve the social participation of users? We know that most citizens of today's world increasingly depend on fast and accessible information exchange technology. Where are the AAC users in this? Are they behind, or will research and development keep the AAC user up to speed (literally)? McNaughton and Bryen (2007) conducted a literature study to analyze this question, and came to the conclusion that there are important questions that are still wide open and unanswered. They suggest that research in the following five areas are critical to advancing the field:

1. *Qualities of face-to-face communication*: As we know, in face-to-face communication, speed is of the essence, and that is where present-day AAC technology is still not where we would want it to be. We will need systems that allow quick access to vocabulary and/or that allow on-the-spot generation of messages.

2. *Distance communication and interconnectivity*: AAC devices should easily connect with cell phone technology. Cell phone technology must be accessible to individuals with limited motor and visual abilities.

3. *Training and support for system use*: Generating messages and introducing yourself (as an AAC user) when you begin a conversation depend on strategies that should in part be learnable. Research can help us to understand what distinguishes successful AAC communicators from less successful ones. What is it that makes some AAC

users easily connect with their partners, and keep them interested and entertained? Is it language skills? Or is it some combination of social skills (charm?)? Or what?

4. *Adapted applications and cognitive tools*: Examples include adapted applications to support access to e-mail, social media, and other Internet functions, switch rapidly between functions (e.g., face-to-face communication and taking notes) and provide cognitive tools (e.g., calendars).

5. *Independent operation, development, and maintenance*: Many AAC users depend heavily on technology. A day without the technology (a day of a breakdown) can be a communicative and personal catastrophe.

The community starts with the family (child with parent, or person with spouse) but extends into the whole family, the friends, the peers, the neighborhood, the classroom, the school, the work environment, the playground, the place of worship (church, synagogue, temple, mosque), the residence, the city council, and more. Will AAC allow a person to function at all of these levels where it is desired?

Blackstone and Hunt-Berg (2003) used the concept of multiple social networks (Figure 12–1) to create an assessment framework that helps to evaluate effectiveness of communication by AAC users in different contexts. They work with the concept of concentric circles with each representing a wider social context.

This framework, which is increasingly used in AAC evaluations and intervention planning, nicely illustrates how communication takes place in several social contexts, each with its own expectations, sets of partners, and challenges. The

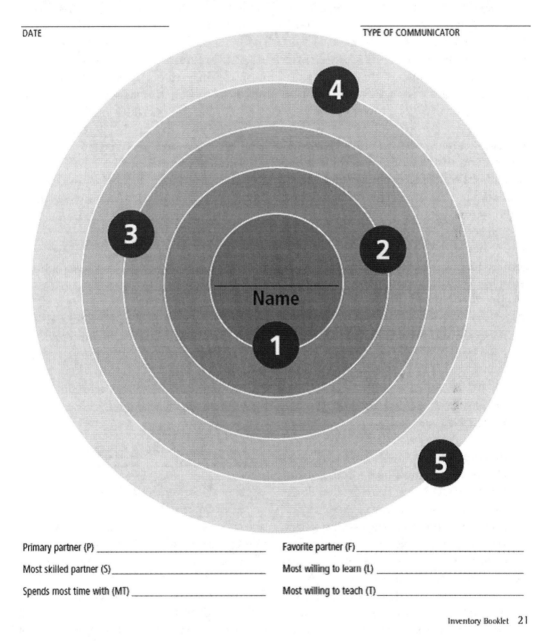

Figure 12–1. Social networks. Reproduced with permission.

framework allows describing how a person's development typically is reflected in an increase in interaction and communicative skills in circles that are more removed from the center. The "circles" are: (1) family, (2) friends, (3) acquaintances, (4) paid workers, and (5) strangers. The growth or development through the circles is not necessarily linear, as a study by Clarke and colleagues (2012) shows. Older children are not necessarily participating at a higher level than younger children. Much depends on the obvious dynamic "interaction between age, level of speech intelligibility, and the perceived effectiveness of the communication aids" (Clarke et al., 2012, p. 49).

A developmental and intervention goal is to obtain *self-determination* (McNaughton, Rackensperger, Wehmeyer, & Wright, 2010), the ability to make choices based on an understanding of self and the ability to set and pursue tactical and strategic life goals.

MULTIPLE CHALLENGES

While one of the ultimate goals of AAC ought to be a maximal participation in social networks, it is clear that individuals who use and need AAC do in fact face multiple challenges when they enter the social circles. We briefly discuss some of the challenges and the possible approaches: (1) attitudes and AAC, (2) AAC in the family, (3) AAC in education, (4) AAC and transitions to adult life, (5) AAC in the workplace, (6) AAC and the development of friendships, (7) communication assistants, (8) AAC users and aging, (9) connections with the world, (10) AAC users' risk of abuse, and (11) AAC users and research.

ATTITUDES AND AAC

How are individuals who use AAC perceived? What do people think about them? And, very importantly, what do AAC users (and their parents and communication partners) think that other people think? When discussing AAC options with adults, this is often a major issue—it is sometimes the main determiner of whether a person will actually adopt a communication device.

Research has indicated that often feelings of discomfort, fear, and insecurity exist along with stereotypes and rejection (Krahé & Altwasser, 2006). Gorenflo and Gorenflo (1997) found that attitudes can be influenced by the perceived discrepancy of the synthetic speech and the AAC user. However, attitudes can change as a result of information. Johnson, Bloomberg, and Iacono (2004) reported that taking a course in AAC led to a significant improvement in undergraduates' attitudes, perception, and willingness to interact with individuals with severe disabilities.

Children's Attitudes

Beck and Dennis (1996) noticed differences between the attitudes of nondisabled boys and girls in fifth grade toward peers who used AAC to communicate. Girls showed a more positive attitude. In this and later studies (Beck, Bock, Thompson, & Kosuwan, 2002; Beck, Fritz, Keller, & Dennis, 2000), they discovered a decrease in positive views both in boys and girls as they progress into middle school. What is it that helps a child to be accepted and liked by his or her peers? As is the case in individuals without a disability, being accepted as a peer and being popular as a child clearly depends on multiple personal and situational factors. Group dynamics play a role. Maybe we should make an effort to make AAC and the children who use AAC more attractive and interesting to their peers. Recently, many have thought that the newer "cooler" devices may somewhat rub off on the child himself. Something like: if you own a fun and cool device, you must be a cool guy yourself. Device developers have come to pay more attention to this potential factor. In an interview Richard Ellenson, one of the developers of a device (the father of a child who needs and uses AAC), states: "The devices at the time were focused on building sentences. To a person in advertising, that doesn't equate to communication. Communication is a much richer notion that involves engaging someone in real time. It involves inflection, prosody, speaking in a language and a voice that people relate to, showing off a sense of coolness, being up to speed on your world" (Holland Bloorview Kids Rehabilitation Hospital, 2009). It has been suggested that the social participation of the AAC user could improve if the vocabulary in the device were more in line with what children in their age-range normally use. Besides a message such as, "How are you doing today?," the child would also have the option to use, "Hey, dude, what's up?" or something along these lines. Would that make a difference? Again, Beck and her associates (Beck, Bock, Thompson, Bowman, & Robbins, 2006) wanted to know the answer to this question. They asked children without a disability in grades 4 and 5 to watch one of two variations of the same videotaped script. The two versions were "formal" and "informal," and differed in how ideas were worded by the AAC users, including "hi, how are you" (formal) ver-

sus "hey, what's up? (informal), "not at all—he was too mean" (formal) versus "gimme a break—he gave me the creeps" (informal), "that scared me" (formal) versus "that freaked me out" (informal), and so on. After watching these videos, the students had to indicate on a rating scale how much they agreed on statements like, "I like children who use AAC," "Children who use AAC scare me," or "I would walk in the school halls with a child who uses AAC." The question is whether the children who had seen the "cool" videotape would show a more positive attitude toward AAC. Interestingly, the results did not indicate any difference in attitude that depended on whether the student had seen the formal or the informal (the cool) video. Attitudes are obviously complex and are not simply modified or altered by one single variable. One other aspect in understanding peer interaction with a child who uses aided AAC is the fact that the dynamics of interaction are different from those between non-AAC users. Clarke and Wilkinson (2008) analyzed dyadic interaction between children with cerebral palsy who used devices and their peers without a disability, and found several breakdowns that were due to difficulties by the nondisabled in grasping the pragmatics of device-based interactions.

AAC AND THE FAMILY

Communication involves interactions between and among many individuals. When there is a problem with communicating a message, that problem is shared both by the communicator and the listener(s). Similarly, all partners also share communication solutions. If I have trouble expressing myself to you, you will have trouble understanding me. If the solution for my problem means that I have to communicate in a different way, it will also mean that you will receive my message in a different way. AAC is a shared phenomenon. Its success (or failure) will be highly determined by whether the communication partners are on board. This is especially the case in young children. Understanding the needs of parents and other family members is crucial for progress. In the first place, these needs are related to feelings of being able to meet present and future communication needs (Angelo, Kokoska, & Jones, 1996). Marshall and Goldbart (2008) conducted semi-structured interviews with the parents or caregivers of 11 children between 3 and 10 years who were AAC users in the United Kingdom. A general conclusion was that parents have a good understanding of their children's needs, functioning, and of the role and potential of AAC.

One must realize that the family should be the first place to look to evaluate the functionality of communication. The family can be regarded as the place where the child needs to learn how to interact with others to survive and to gain a level of happy and effective functioning. Granlund and his colleagues (Granlund, Bjorck-Åkesson, Wilder, & Ylven, 2008) analyzed the existing studies and concluded that AAC work in the family should focus on the quality and the quantity of participation. Active participation should be the goal. Use of AAC is one of the means to get to this goal. Iacono (2003) analyzed all the AAC intervention studies published in the *AAC* journal from 1985 to 2000. She used the International Classification of Functioning, Disability, and Health (ICF) as proposed by the World Health Organization (Raghavendra, Bornman, Granlund, & Bjorck-Åkesson, 2007).

The majority of the studies tried to describe the type of device or method that was provided, or focused on how AAC (the device, the method) was used, but did not go into the social participation. In their literature study, Granlund and collaborators stated that family studies in AAC would be most fruitful if they could invest in:

1. *Determining the effectiveness of different AAC methods:* Which of all the methods is most likely to work given the entire configuration of factors (both in the child or adult AAC user, the communication partners, and the environment) that are present. It should be remembered that studies of effectiveness are often conducted by researchers in well-controlled conditions (as they should be). When you want to transfer the method from the lab to the home situation, it will be extremely important to instruct, model, and guide the parents and others (siblings can be essential) in how to interact and serve as effective communication partners.

2. *Translating the research evidence into family conditions:* Transposing an intervention to a family is a complicated matter. Not all families will "respond" to the same suggested intervention in the same way. Margalit, Al-Yagon, and Kleitman (2006) described types of families with different characteristics that affect the way they respond to family intervention. Factors that play a role include cohesiveness of the family, ability to cope with parenting stress, general mood, and family adaptability. It is important to recognize and anticipate that the same method used with a child or adult with a similar cognitive and communication profile may not yield

the same results because the family responds in a different way.

Things differ from family to family. Every family has its own culture, and every family is part of one or more broader cultures. McCord and Soto (2004) noticed important attitudinal differences during a series of interviews with Mexican-American parents of AAC users. The father of a 14-year-old boy, who had been living in the United States for 10 years, had this to say: "With me, he has always communicated. We don't need a machine to tell me what he wants to say. Yes, he can glance in a direction and I can follow his eyes, like a mother does with her infant. For someone who doesn't believe in that, like many people from the USA, they don't trust themselves to know what he says or they don't trust him. They need the technology. And he can do it that way for them." (p. 217) We are in need of more research that helps us to understand all the cultural aspects of the use of AAC. Every culture has implicit assumptions and values concerning how people relate to each other in different situations, starting with the family. For example, Johnston and Wong (2002) discuss the differences in cultural perceptions on how parents could and should provide language support through interaction between Chinese and Western North American families. Clinicians should recognize the values and priorities that exist within the culture. However, the authors also suggest that sometimes parents can be asked to put aside reluctances toward a type of intervention that might feel culturally awkward to them. The authors state, "Educators and speech-language pathologists may help families override cultural norms (e.g., accept the use of sign) by explicitly identifying such practices as extraordinary, but important,

parental responses to a child's learning needs" (p. 923).

Finally, everyone knows that it will not be sufficient just to tell the parents once what they are supposed to do and expect that the method will be implemented. Parents—and all family members for that matter—need to obtain ownership of the adopted method. It needs to be "their" intervention, not the intervention that they do following instructions from a speech-language pathologist or a researcher. The role of the professional is to support and be attentive for maintenance (i.e., ensure that the method becomes an integral part of the family's daily operating style).

In the end, all parents and their children follow a unique and challenging path, exploring avenues, dealing with uncertainties, frustrations, but also hope and moments of happiness (Rummel-Hudson, 2008).

AAC IN EDUCATION

During all formative years of life, people's perspective on their own place in the community (leadership, ways to make friendships, ways to interact, ways to solve differences in opinion) is highly influenced by models and opportunities. It is evident that much of the initial education will take place in the family and school. Education in a more general sense is a community process. Involving children, including those who use AAC, in the community outside the school and the family at a young age, might provide critical experiences and a critical learning environment. One of the advantages is that social learning and participation can have its free course, without being strictly guided by an educational plan with preset objectives and methods. Children who are AAC users can and should get involved in local activities, organized by the church, the library, and other agencies. Batorowicz, McDougall, and Shepherd (2006) studied the possibility of including children who are AAC users as full participants. They describe how children who are AAC users got involved in a *Story Time* and a *Dress Up and Drama* project. Programs such as those turn out to be very beneficial for all partners involved: The children who use AAC are recognized and valued as unique contributors. They also have new opportunities to interact and communicate naturally in a community event. For the nondisabled children, a new world opens up too. The adults (e.g., librarians) reported that they learned things they would be able to apply to other groups (things they never did with nondisabled children, but would be fun to do), and they felt appreciated through attention and media coverage. They also mentioned that their perception of children who use AAC had changed dramatically.

Inclusiveness

Succeeding at *school* involves different aspects. We can talk about academic success, but we also need to talk about personal success. Academic success relates to achieving skills and learning objectives, and is measurable by assessing skills and learning objectives that are achieved. Personal success relates more to a sense of social well-being that is reinforced by an environment of student peers. In other words, how well is the AAC user accepted, loved, admired, avoided, and so on, by the student peers? It depends.

From the Beck et al. 2006 study, we learn that attitudes of peers toward AAC users are not always as positive as we would like them to be.

How inclusive can and should schools be when pursuing the best possible educational results for the students? Inclusion is certainly not always as easy as one would wish. In their interview study with parents, Marshall and Goldbart (2008) indicate that the communication limitations really pose a barrier to inclusion: "It is so very hard . . . that stops children like Hannah from having friends" and "When they play 'school' she misses out physically . . . she is part of it but she does miss out on the banter" (p. 90).

Hunt-Berg (2005) reported on an archival study of alumni of the Bridge School, an educational program located outside San Francisco. The school is unique in that it has a strong focus on developing communicative competence for students who rely on AAC. The students are given intensive AAC services and training during a period of their school career, before going back to their own school district. Providing such an intensive program leads to a high percentage of success in terms of independence and further inclusive functioning. However, school inclusion is not always achieved in every case, as parents make decisions based on a combination of factors.

Talking about inclusion, it is worth asking how well children with AAC needs are received when they walk into the school. Do teachers and other team members regard them as a welcome student, a challenge, a burden, or what? Bailey and her colleagues (Bailey, Stoner, Parette, & Angell, 2006) looked at just that. They interviewed a team of six special education teachers and one speech-language pathologist. This team appeared to have responded to the challenge by clearly formulating the areas that matter for success and for effective teaching of students who are AAC users. They identified four main areas that are critical: (1) the student's communicative competence, (2) the existing barriers (time constraints, limitations inherent to the specific device that the student uses, and incongruence with the parents/guardians (Incongruence refers to a lack of cooperation or differences in perspectives on the AAC needs between the school team and the parents), (3) the instructional benefits (increased independence, effective teaching, the use of the device across settings), and (4) facilitators (positive parental involvement, ease of use of the AAC system). This study gives a picture that indicates that successful use of AAC in the schools can be a reality if the team is fully on board and if the team is willing and given the resources to address the challenges.

Of course, including children who are AAC users into a classroom can be an educational challenge if one has not done it before and if one doesn't know what to expect and what the answers are. All parties involved may feel insecure about how to go about it. Kent-Walsh and Light (2003) conducted interviews with general education teachers about their experiences with one or more children who are using AAC. One major barrier is clearly a general feeling of not knowing "how to do this." Teachers, as well as their supervisors, may have no idea what to expect, how to organize, plan, and how to deal with behavior-related problems. In describing how she found out that she would have a person who was an AAC user in her class, one teacher said: "It was a shock. The door opened, as I was call-ing off the attendance to make sure all my students were there on the first day, and she was wheeled in" (p. 112).

The authors describe the following three team-related components of successful inclusion, as they were indicated by the participants in the study: (a) effective team communication and collaboration; (b) adequate classroom support provided by educational assistants with training, skills, and dedication to the inclusive education of students who use AAC; and (c) appropriate general education teacher training and preparation time (p. 120). Good classroom inclusion will be highly dependent on both teacher preparation/skills and good targeted functioning of the teacher teams.

How do we go about ensuring that children with AAC needs get the best educational strategies and supports in the classroom? Grether and Sickman (2008) suggest that the Response to Intervention (RTI) approach may offer the best possible conceptual and organizational framework to meet AAC users' needs. They propose a three-tier approach consisting of initially identifying students who are at risk (tier 1), providing the children with in-classroom interventions (tier 2), and, in case of insufficient response with the tier 2 intervention, the provision of additional aids (tier 3). When it comes to children with AAC needs, the speech-language pathologist will often be the one who plays a key role in feeding information and suggestions to the team, and coordinating the work in the different tiers. Someone will need to address issues about how to use a device or other nonspeech communication aids (including manual signs) in a classroom environment in such a way that it will not disrupt the flow of events, and how to include the student in class discussions, groups, and activities, so that he or she can interact in the time available. This depends not only on the student but also on the opportunities provided and the way the teacher structures the class, taking into account the student's use of AAC. As everywhere, in the classroom, successful communication and functioning is dependent on several variables. Carter (2003) explored the impact of styles of functioning such as *spontaneity* (defined as whether behavior is elicited by internal controllable factors or not) and suggests that such personal characteristics should be taken into account when planning and predicting the need for intervention.

Universal Design for Learning

Universal Design of Learning (UDL; Dalton, 2012; Pisha & Coyne, 2001) is an approach to organizing educational materials and experiences in such a way that learners who have differing learning styles can all benefit from it. Depending on developmental, academic, and personal cognitive and sensory characteristics, one learner may respond better to one type of exposure while another learner may benefit more from another way of presenting the information. If information is accessible and can be manipulated in different modalities, learners can find which configuration of information leads to the best learning results for them. Multimodality, a principle that we have discussed in other chapters as one of the keys why AAC can work for many learners, can also be considered to be a more general didactic principle: present information in many formats (modalities) and allow the learners to take advantage from modalities that work best for them. Good educa-

tional approaches for students, who use and need AAC, are likely to be also effective for non-AAC users.

POST-HIGH SCHOOL

Post-secondary school education is different for everyone, as it implies a greater autonomy and an increased perspective on choices toward a meaningful adult life. The type of service at this level is usually different from what the student was used to, and it will require the ability to take initiative and be proactive (Horn & May, 2010). Meaningfulness of life is determined by many factors, including work but also leisure. Although there are unquestionably barriers for AAC users to have access to creative use of leisure time (financial, practical), solutions exist to overcome these (AAC device use, personal care assistant, social networking; Dattilo et al., 2008). Recreation is an exceptionally powerful source for social participation, social networking, natural and spontaneous practice and improvement of communication, and education of the public about AAC and AAC users (Dattilo, Benedek-Wood, & McLeod, 2010).

However, the post-school experiences are often not so positive and sometimes outright discouraging. In a qualitative study with eight participants in Canada, Hamm and Mirenda (2006) found that a discrepancy existed between communication skills that had been taught and trained during the school years and the reality post-school. Some participants were "stuck where they were" without the psychological or material resources to take initiative, identify their life barriers, and address them (Hamm & Mirenda, 2006).

TRANSITIONS TO ADULT LIFE

How do AAC users see their future? What are the self-expectations? Expectations and a view of the future do not develop in a vacuum. Everybody's perception and hopes are influenced and shaped by parental and teacher expectations, and by models—or sometimes by the lack of models. Do young AAC users have access or knowledge of other successful AAC users?

Transition to adult life will require practical and logistic arrangements such as a place to live and health care (Balandin & Waller, 2010), a continuation of AAC related service (Ball, Stading, & Hazelrigg, 2010), besides psychological and social growth plans, including meaningful activities, the development of a circle of friends, and relationship skills (McNaughton & Kennedy, 2010).

AAC IN THE WORKPLACE

Transition to work is not easy and may need to be accompanied by an employment preparation and guidance program (Cohen, Bryen, & Carey, 2003). Since 1991, an organization called SHOUT has been organizing the biennial Pittsburgh Employment Conference. The conference is unique as it is directed at individuals who use AAC and who are employed and play a leadership role. It shows what a tremendous difference AAC can make. In the era that AAC did not yet exist or was not readily available, employment was simply not even something that would be considered. That was only one generation ago —or less. Therefore, it is impressive to see individuals who are AAC users and who

are active in the workforce, sometimes as self-employed workers or, in most cases, as part-time or full-time employees.

However, the reality is that the number of AAC users who are employed still constitutes a minority. Blackstone estimated in 1993 that 85% of the AAC users are unemployed (Blackstone, 1993). What is it that brings some of the AAC users to successful employment while the majority of them never get there? Obviously, it is a multitude of factors that work together. Meyer, Loncke, and Goldkamp (2008) looked at archives of a vocational training (Woodrow Wilson Rehabilitation Center in Fishersville, VA) center for individuals who were AAC users and, in hindsight, tried to determine what have been the most powerful forces in driving a person toward employment (or preventing it). Through the archive study, the researchers were able to identify the main barriers in finishing vocational training and progressing to the workforce. The barriers included: (1) communication barriers (slow or reluctant use of AAC, interpersonal communication, expressive communication), (2) limited academic skills, including lack of literacy, and (3) slow work speed and insufficiently appropriate work attitudes and work habits (i.e., being timely, anticipate what will be needed for a task, etc.). Other barriers included lack of attention to detail, concentration problems, limited work experience and knowledge, and work energy and stamina. These factors need to be taken into consideration if one wishes for vocational training to be effective (i.e., if one really wants to have more participation of AAC users in employment settings). Bryen and colleagues drew similar conclusions from interviews with employers of individuals who used AAC: the level of education is important, but skills such as time management, problem solving, and basic technology are also highly regarded (Bryen, Potts, & Carey, 2007).

We live in a society where the work contribution of a person to the community (through some kind of work—paid or unpaid) is an essential factor in societal and personal esteem. Not being part of the working and creative forces of a community increases the risk of self-depreciation. In 2009, during a time of economic crisis in the United States and worldwide, the Pittsburgh Employment Conference chose as its central theme: "Employment: Overcoming Depression and Loneliness"—the theme of the conference reveals a major concern of this group who often are struck by a double blow of being communicatively disabled (with all the challenges, prejudices, and stereotypes) and being underemployed (again, with all the challenges, prejudices, and stereotypes).

For individuals who do find employment and are successful in it, there still remain considerable problems. "Getting your 'wheel' in the door," as McNaughton, Light, and Arnold (2002) put it, is not an easy accomplishment. These authors conducted focus group discussions with eight individuals with cerebral palsy who use AAC and were employed full-time. This study sheds light both on the benefits and the challenges of employment for AAC users. Benefits include the salary, the achievement of success, positive impact on self-esteem, and contact with other people. There are also many challenges: negative attitudes of society and employers toward individuals with disabilities, low expectations from others, inappropriate education, lack of funding for assistive technology, transportation difficulties, and fatigue from full-time work.

McNaughton, Light, and Gulla (2003) also conducted a survey with employers and coworkers of individuals who use AAC. The picture they got from this perspective was equally interesting. Employers and coworkers who do work with individuals who use AAC experience on a daily basis the benefits and the challenges. From an employer's perspective, hiring a person who uses AAC can: (1) be personally rewarding, (2) have positive effects on other employees, (3) lead to high quality work performance by the employee, (4) create the possibility to obtain grants, (5) assure loyalty of the employee, and (6) occasionally provide you with the ability to fill a "hard to fill" position (p. 240).

The discussion with all parties has led to a remarkable list of recommendations to make employment a possibility and more successful. Of course, successful employment will start with expectations and good education. Successful employment will depend on the contribution of many stakeholders, starting with the AAC users themselves.

AAC AND THE DEVELOPMENT OF FRIENDSHIPS

Cooper, Balandin, and Trembath (2009) published an article under the title "The Loneliness Experiences of Young Adults with Cerebral Palsy who use Alternative and Augmentative Communication." They conducted in-depth interviews with individuals with cerebral palsy who were AAC users. Although having AAC was widely recognized by all as a powerful phenomenon that provided them a great deal of independence, at the same time the interviews reflected problems such as lack of privacy, difficulty to have friends who have the time, the skills and the willingness to communicate with an AAC user, and limited literacy skills. Many things in life, that nondisabled people take for granted, are not readily available to disabled individuals who need AAC. For example, take the telephone. One of the participants in the study mentioned "It takes such a long time for me to have a telephone conversation . . . I hardly ever talk to my friends on the phone" (p. 160). Not being able to use the telephone intensifies loneliness in our society. Or, even more in today's world: the computer and the use of Internet. One of the participants spelled on her alphabet board "n-o-t e-v-e-r-y-o-n-e h-a-s a c-o-m-p-u-t-e-r" (p. 160).

COMMUNICATION ASSISTANTS

Assistants, whether they are paid or not, find themselves in the role of connectors and interpreters between the person with communication needs and the environment. Hemsley and Balandin (2004) describe how unpaid assistants constantly are fighting disabling attitudes in medical personnel in the hospital, which is reflected in such habits as not directing questions and information to the persons with communication needs but to their assistants. Caregivers and attendants report that they consider themselves to be models of how to interact with a person with AAC needs. Communication assistants perform a complex set of tasks. Their effectiveness can improve communication between AAC users and all members of the wider community (Collier, McGhie-Richmond, & Self, 2010; Collier & Self, 2010).

AGING

Balandin and Morgen (2001) have also focused on the challenges of aging for individuals with AAC. For the entire population, aging comes with increased risk of loss of visual acuity—often one of the senses that is crucial for the AAC solution (seeing the device is important), less mobility, and frequently fewer financial resources. However, for individuals with disabilities, the "cumulative impact of aging, cerebral palsy, and AAC raises many questions for which we do not have answers at this time. This is partly due to the fact that, to date, there are few augmented communicators with cerebral palsy who are in or are approaching their senior years" (p. 107). Unfortunately, the results of Balandin's work are somewhat depressing. Often the medical caregivers do not understand the disabling condition well enough to appreciate the importance of the alternative forms of communication. They may not see how the very process of aging can be a threat to the AAC solutions that have been developed over time. The study also revealed that many AAC users are not used to talk about their health issues with medical professionals. The quality of life of aging AAC users needs to be taken seriously.

CONNECTIONS WITH THE WORLD

Today's interconnected world offers opportunities for individuals who rely on AAC to interact with virtual everybody on the globe (DeRuyter, McNaughton, Caves, Bryen, & Williams, 2007). Has the Internet opened up opportunities for AAC users that did not exist beforehand? It certainly has. However, an important question relates to whether AAC users have the same access and facility of communication as anybody. Bryen, Heake, Semenuk, and Segal (2010) point out that navigating the web requires a way of reading information that may not be as accessible for individuals who rely on AAC (e.g., graphic symbols) and who may need accessibility enhancement tools.

RISK OF ABUSE

One of the sad realities of life is the fact that individuals with little or no functional speech are at a greater risk of becoming victims of abuse. It is only in the past 10 years that our workers, victims, and psychologists have demanded attention for this problem (Bryen, Carey, & Frantz, 2003).

In a review of the data, Huer (2006) put some statistics on this problem. Individuals with developmental disabilities are four to five times more likely to become victims of crime. The risks are the highest for sexual assault (10.7 times as high) and robbery (12.7 times as high). Also, there is a high probability of repeat victimization. Fifty percent of women with developmental disabilities who had been sexually assaulted had been assaulted 10 or more times.

The underlying reason why these individuals are so easily victimized is clear: Victims with developmental disabilities are frequently invisible because they cannot report their offenders. The crimes often remain unreported, or the reports are discredited.

For the longest time, parents and professionals have not been aware of this

problem. In the past few years, there have been efforts to better prepare children (and adults) without functional speech: (1) to recognize and interpret behaviors that are inappropriate, (2) to learn how to say "no," how to protest, and certainly (3) to report unwanted behaviors from others. Educators must set goals that include awareness of a person's own dignity, and a person's right to be respected, protected, and defended (Hingsburger, 2010).

AAC USERS AND RESEARCH

As part of a general movement in several fields of applied research, several voices (augmented or not) have expressed the need to give a more important role and position to individuals who use AAC in different aspects of AAC research. As in most fields, the researchers themselves are those who determine the research agenda (i.e., the research questions, the goals of what is needed). Balandin and Raghavendra (1999) formulated a series of interesting ideas that would lead to more participation of AAC users in research. For example, they suggest that one should work with a research steering group that can function as a sounding board to inform users and the public, as well as generate ideas to increase the social validity and relevance of the research. Many see the growing participation of AAC users in research projects as part of an empowerment movement. "Nothing About Me Without Me" is the title of a book chapter written about this principle by Bersani (1999). The point is to establish a culture of research that is respectful and keeps the person who needs AAC at the center of all research endeavors. Bersani

(1999, p. 288) makes a number of policy suggestions including:

- Development of a policy statement to encourage the participation of consumers in every stage of AAC research.
- Encouragement of authors to include information about the level and variety of consumer participation in manuscripts submitted for publication.
- Offering of training sessions to prepare augmented speakers for new roles in research.

Being an AAC user affects a person's personal and social life every single day. It is important that professionals understand this. The impact of the need for AAC should not be reduced to a mere problem of information exchange through message formulation.

POINTS TO REMEMBER

- The way AAC and communication modalities are used differs depending on the needs of the situation and the familiarity of the communication partners.
- Universal Design of Learning is an approach that attempts to present educational materials and experiences in such a way that multiple styles of cognitive and linguistic information processing are accommodated. Such a philosophy agrees with the basic principles of AAC.
- Attitudes toward and inclusion of students who use AAC are influenced by multiple factors, including the

perceived discrepancy of the synthetic speech and the AAC user. But attitudes can change by providing information and by increasing participation.

- Adoption and integration of AAC methods in the family depends on multiple factors such as cohesiveness of the family, ability to cope with parenting stress, general mood, family adaptability, and cultural openness toward AAC methods and AAC related technology.
- As education responds to the needs of students who use AAC, they are more likely to have positive post-high school experiences and stronger expectations and attitudes toward integration in the workplace.
- Post-school transitions and integration in the workplace of individuals who use AAC pose many challenges often due to low (self-) expectations.
- The social life of individuals using AAC can pose many challenges such as the lack of privacy, lack of opportunities to make friends and build relationships, and limited literacy skills.
- Special attention needs to be paid to the aging generation of AAC users who can experience a variety of health problems that risk to complicate social life and even the AAC solutions that worked before.

REFERENCES

Angelo, D., Kokoska, S., & Jones, S. (1996). Family perspective on augmentative and alternative communication: Families of adolescents and young adults. *AAC: Augmentative and Alternative Communication, 12*(1), 13–22.

Bailey, R., Stoner, J., Parette, H., Jr., & Angell, M. (2006). AAC team perceptions: Augmentative and alternative communication device use. *Education and Training in Developmental Disabilities, 41*(2), 139–154.

Balandin, S., & Morgan, J. (2001). Preparing for the future: Aging and alternative and augmentative communication. *AAC: Augmentative and Alternative Communication, 17*(2), 99–108.

Balandin, S., & Raghavendra, P. (1999). Challenging oppression: Augmented communicators' involvement in AAC research. In F. Loncke, J. Clibbens, H. Arvidson, & L. Lloyd (Eds.), *Augmentative and alternative communication: New directions in research and practice* (pp. 262–277). London, UK: Whurr.

Balandin, S., & Waller, A. (2010). Medical and health transitions for young adults who use AAC. In D. McNaughton & D. Beukelman (Eds.), *Transition strategies for adolescents and young adults who use AAC* (pp. 181–198). Baltimore, MD: Paul H. Brookes.

Ball, L., Stading, K., & Hazelrigg, D. (2010). AAC considerations during the transition to adult life. In D. McNaughton & D. Beukelman (Eds.), *Transition strategies for adolescents and young adults who use AAC* (pp. 201–217). Baltimore, MD: Paul H. Brookes.

Batorowicz, B., McDougall, S., & Shepherd, T. A. (2006). AAC and community partnerships: The participation path to community inclusion. *Augmentative and Alternative Communication, 22*(3), 178–195.

Beck, A., Bock, S., Thompson, J., Bowman, L., & Robbins, S. (2006). Is awesome really awesome? How the inclusion of informal terms on an AAC device influences children's attitudes toward peers who use AAC. *Research in Developmental Disabilities, 27*(1), 56–69.

Beck, A., Bock, S., Thompson, J., & Kosuwan, K. (2002). Influence of communicative competence and augmentative and alternative communication technique on children's attitudes toward a peer who uses AAC. *AAC: Augmentative and Alternative Communication, 18*(4), 217–227.

Beck, A., & Dennis, M. (1996). Attitudes of children toward a similar-aged child who uses augmentative communication. *AAC: Augmentative and Alternative Communication, 12*(2), 78–87.

Beck, A., Fritz, H., Keller, A., & Dennis, M. (2000). Attitudes of school-aged children toward their peers who use augmentative and alternative communication. *AAC: Augmentative and Alternative Communication, 16*(1), 13–26.

Bersani, H. (1999). Nothing about me without me: A proposal for participatory action research in AAC. In F. Loncke, J. Clibbens, H. Arvidson, & L. Lloyd (Eds.), *Augmentative and alternative communication: New directions in research and practice* (pp. 278–289). London, UK: Whurr.

Blackstone, S. (1993). For consumers: What do you want to be when you grow up? *Augmentative Communication News, 6*(4), 1–2.

Blackstone, S., & Hunt-Berg, M. (2003). *Social networks: A communication inventory for individuals with complex communication needs and their communication partners manual.* Monterey, CA: Augmentative Communication.

Bryen, D. N., Carey, A., & Frantz, B. (2003). Ending the silence: Adults who use augmentative communication and their experiences as victims of crimes. *AAC: Augmentative and Alternative Communication, 19*(2), 125–134.

Bryen, D., Heake, G., Semenuk, A., & Segal, M. (2010). Improving web access for individuals who rely on augmentative and alternative communication. *AAC: Augmentative and Alternative Communication, 26*(1), 21–29.

Bryen, D., Potts, B., & Carey, A. C. (2007). So you want to work? What employers say about job skills, recruitment and hiring employees who rely on AAC. *AAC: Augmentative and Alternative Communication, 23*(2), 126–139.

Carter, M. (2003). Communicative spontaneity of children with high support needs who use augmentative and alternative communication systems I: Classroom spontaneity, mode, and function. *AAC: Augmentative and Alternative Communication, 19*(3), 141–154.

Clarke, M., Newton, C., Petrides, K., Griffiths, T., Lysley, A., & Price, K. (2012). An examination of relations between participation, communication and age in children with complex communication needs. *AAC: Augmentative and Alternative Communication, 28*(1), 44–51.

Clarke, M., & Wilkinson, R. (2008). Interaction between children with cerebral palsy and their peers 2: Understanding initiated VOCA-mediated turns. *AAC: Augmentative and Alternative Communication, 24*(1), 3–15.

Cohen, K., Bryen, D., & Carey, A. (2003). Augmentative communication employment training and supports (ACETS). *AAC: Augmenta-*

tive and Alternative Communication, 19(3), 199–206.

Collier, B., McGhie-Richmond, D., & Self, H. (2010). Exploring communication assistants as an option for increasing communication access to communities for people who use augmentative communication. *AAC: Augmentative and Alternative Communication, 26*(1), 48–59.

Collier, B., & Self, H. (2010). Preparing youth who use AAC to communicate with their personal assistant. In D. McNaughton & D. Beukelman (Eds.), *Transition strategies for adolescents and young adults who use AAC* (pp. 163–180). Baltimore, MD: Paul H. Brookes.

Cooper, L., Balandin, S., & Trembath, D. (2009). The loneliness experiences of young adults with cerebral palsy who use alternative and augmentative communication. *AAC: Augmentative and Alternative Communication, 25*(3), 154–164.

Dalton, E. M. (2012). The assessment of young children through the lens of universal design for learning (UDL). *Forum on Public Policy.*

Dattilo, J., Benedek-Wood, E., & McLeod, L. (2010). "Activity brings community into our lives": Recreation, leisure, and community participation for individuals who use AAC. In D. McNaughton & D. Beukelman (Eds.), *Transition strategies for adolescents and young adults who use AAC* (pp. 131–144). Baltimore, MD: Paul H. Brookes.

Dattilo, J., Estrella, G., Estrella, L. J., Light, J., McNaughton, D., & Seabury, M. (2008). "I have chosen to live life abundantly": Perceptions of leisure by adults who use augmentative and alternative communication. *AAC: Augmentative and Alternative Communication, 24*(1), 16–28.

DeRuyter, F., McNaughton, D., Caves, K., Bryen, D. N., & Williams, M. (2007). Enhancing AAC connections with the world. *AAC: Augmentative and Alternative Communication, 23*(3), 258–270.

Ellenson, R. *Seen and heard. Interview with Richard Ellenson.* Retrieved May 29, 2013, from http://www.hollandbloorview.ca/bloomwinter 2009/Bloom/Seen_and_heard.html

Gorenflo, D., & Gorenflo, C. (1997). Effects of synthetic speech, gender, and perceived similarity on attitudes toward the augmented communicator. *AAC: Augmentative and Alternative Communication, 13*(2), 87–91.

Granlund, M., Bjorck-Åkesson, E., Wilder, J., & Ylven, R. (2008). AAC interventions for children in a family environment: Implementing evidence in practice. *AAC: Augmentative and Alternative Communication, 24*(3), 207–219.

Grether, S., & Sickman, L. (2008). AAC and RTI: Building classroom-based strategies for every child in the classroom. *Seminars in Speech and Language, 29*(2), 155–163.

Hamm, B., & Mirenda, P. (2006). Post-school quality of life for individuals with developmental disabilities who use AAC. *AAC: Augmentative and Alternative Communication, 22*(2), 134–147.

Hemsley, B., & Balandin, S. (2004). Without AAC: The stories of unpaid carers of adults with cerebral palsy and complex communication needs in hospital. *AAC: Augmentative and Alternative Communication, 20*(4), 243–258.

Hingsburger, D. (2010). The language of love. Sexuality and people who use AAC. In D. McNaughton & D. Beukelman (Eds.), *Transition strategies for adolescents and young adults who use AAC* (pp. 145–160). Baltimore, MD: Paul H. Brookes.

Holland Bloorview Kids Rehabilitation Hospital. (2009). *Giving Thomas a voice that's cool. Interview with Richard Ellenson.* Retrieved from http://bloom-parentingkidswithdisabilities .blogspot.com/2009/10/giving-thomas-voice -thats-cool.html

Horn, C., & May, R. (2010). Post-high school transition supports and programs in postsecondary education for young adults who use AAC. In D. McNaughton & D. Beukelman (Eds.), *Transition strategies for adolescents and young adults who use AAC* (pp. 93–110). Baltimore, MD: Paul H. Brookes.

Huer, M. (2006). *AAC: Awareness of risk of victimization.* ISAAC Biennial Conference, Dusseldorf, Germany.

Hunt-Berg, M. (2005). The bridge school: Educational inclusion outcomes over 15 years. *AAC: Augmentative and Alternative Communication, 21*(2), 116–131.

Iacono, T. (2003). The evidence base in augmentative and alternative communication. In S. Reily, A. Perry, & J. Douglas (Eds.), *Evidence practice in speech pathology* (pp. 288–313). London, UK: Whurr.

Johnson, H., Bloomberg, K., & Iacono, T. (2004). Attitudes towards and willingness to work with people disabilities: Potential impact of a course in augmentative and alternative communication (AAC) [Abstract]. *Journal of Intellectual Disability Research, 48*(4–5), 354.

Johnston, J. R., & Wong, M. A. (2002). Cultural differences in beliefs and practices concerning talk to children. *Journal of Speech, Language and Hearing Research, 45*(5), 916.

Kent-Walsh, J., & Light, J. C. (2003). General education teachers' experiences with inclusion of students who use augmentative and alternative communication. *AAC: Augmentative and Alternative Communication, 19*(2), 104–124.

Krahé, B., & Altwasser, C. (2006). Changing negative attitudes towards persons with physical disabilities: An experimental intervention. *Journal of Community and Applied Social Psychology, 16*(1), 59–69.

Margalit, M., Al-Yagon, M., & Kleitman, T. (2006). Family subtyping and early intervention. *Journal of Policy and Practice in Intellectual Disabilities, 3*(1), 33–41.

Marshall, J., & Goldbart, J. (2008). "Communication is everything I think." Parenting a child who needs augmentative and alternative communication. *International Journal of Language and Communication Disorders, 43*(1), 77–98.

McCord, M., & Soto, G. (2004). Perceptions of AAC: An ethnographic investigation of Mexican-American families. *AAC: Augmentative and Alternative Communication, 20*(4), 209–227.

McNaughton, D., & Bryen, D. N. (2007). AAC technologies to enhance participation and access to meaningful societal roles for adolescents and adults with developmental disabilities who require AAC. *AAC: Augmentative and Alternative Communication, 23*(3), 217–229.

McNaughton, D., & Kennedy, P. (2010). Supporting successful transitions to adult life for individuals who use AAC. In D. McNaughton & D. Beukelman (Eds.), *Transition strategies for adolescents and young adults who use AAC* (pp. 3–15). Baltimore, MD: Paul H. Brookes.

McNaughton, D., Light, J., & Arnold, K. B. (2002). "Getting your wheel in the door": Successful full-time employment experiences of individuals with cerebral palsy who use augmentative and alternative communication. *AAC: Augmentative and Alternative Communication, 18*(2), 59–76.

McNaughton, D., Light, J., & Gulla, S. (2003). Opening up a "whole new world": Employer and co-worker perspectives on working with individuals who use augmentative and alternative communication. *AAC: Augmentative and Alternative Communication, 19*(4), 235–253.

McNaughton, D., Rackensperger, T., Wehmeyer, M., & Wright, S. (2010). Self-determination and young adults who use AAC. In D. McNaughton & D. Beukelman (Eds.), *Transition strategies for adolescents and young adults who use AAC* (pp. 17–32). Baltimore, MD: Paul H. Brookes.

Meyer, L., Loncke, F., & Goldkamp, J. (2008, 26 September). *Factors contributing to success of failure in vocational evaluation by users of augmentative and alternative communication devices.* Poster presented at the 2nd annual Clinical Augmentative and Alternative Communication Research Conference, Charlottesville, VA.

Pisha, B., & Coyne, P. (2001). Smart from the start. *Remedial & Special Education, 22*(4), 197–203.

Raghavendra, P., Bornman, J., Granlund, M., & Bjorck-Åkesson, E. (2007). The World Health Organization's International Classification of Functioning, Disability and Health: Implications for clinical and research practice in the field of augmentative and alternative communication. *Augmentative and Alternative Communication, 23*(4), 349–361.

Rummel-Hudson, R. (2008). *Schuyler's monster. A father's journey with his wordless daughter.* New York, NY: St. Martin's Griffin.

CHAPTER 13

The AAC Experience

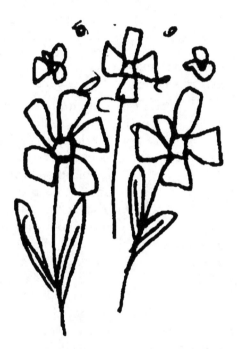

WHAT DOES IT MEAN TO BE AN AAC USER?

Is there something unique about being an AAC user? Would an AAC user be the same if he or she had not been provided with AAC?

In 2000, the International Society for Augmentative and Alternative Communication published a book "Beneath the Surface" (Williams & Krezman, 2000), a bundle of poetry and graphic artwork, exclusively written and made by AAC users. The message of this book was clearly to allow and invite the reader to look beyond the fact that the contributors were AAC users and discover the world of feelings, hopes, frustrations, dreams, certainties, and uncertainties that every human being has. It is not surprising that a condition such as being an AAC user is something that will resonate in the artful expressions of a person.

Consider this poem by Carole Janow (In Williams & Krezman, 2000, p. 78):

Is there a life after speech?
Sometimes late at night
In the silence of my room
I think not

The world is made up of words
Words I cannot utter
Words that no one understands
Conversations only to myself

How can I live without them
It's like being sentenced to die
Everyday is a struggle no one knows
A loneliness only I can feel

For without speech I am disconnected
and apart

In a publication of the French chapter of the International Society for Augmentative and Alternative Communication, I found this little poem, written by an anonymous AAC user:

On m'a pris tous mes gestes
On m'a pris tous les mots
Mais il m'est resté tout le reste
Et tout est beau

(My gestures have been taken away
My words have been taken away
But I still have all the rest
And all is beautiful)

The alternative forms and ways of communicating are often the most salient characteristics for observers. People who use AAC tend to be identified with AAC. In the past 20 years, the "People First" movement has emphasized that it is wrong to talk about "the blind" or "the deaf," but that one should recognize, in terminology, that they are in the first place people (as anyone) with a characteristic (deafness, blindness, etc.; Folkins, 2013). The same should be true for individuals who are AAC users. Nevertheless, the use of AAC is still, for many, such a new phenomenon that one tends to forget that there is a person behind the communication device. A British man with cerebral palsy who is using AAC told me about

what happened when he accompanied his wife to the hospital when she was about to deliver their first baby. For a long time, he had thought he would never become a father, but now here the moment was. Becoming a father and being part of a family of three: that was all that was on his mind and all he wanted to think and talk about. However, when the doctor saw and heard him use his speech-generating communication device, he was very interested in . . . the device. The doctor was fascinated by this machine and ignored the excitement and the happiness of the soon-to-be-father, and bombarded him with questions about the technology of the device. The device had such a tremendous effect on how he perceived his communication partner that he tended to forget that his professional attention should be in line with the emotional experience of the couple who were to become parents.

The communication device stood between the two communication partners and colored the communicative interaction. It is true that communication is a shared phenomenon. Having a communication problem or disorder is never something purely individual. If my communication is difficult because I speak slow and unclear, everybody who will be my communication partner will experience the slowness and lack of clarity.

Therefore, it is very clear that the need for augmented communication has a profound effect on how others see AAC users, how they see themselves, and how their life unfolds. When we consider how communication is the motor that feeds development, cognition, social networking, it is no wonder that it does permeate in the way individuals think and feel about themselves, and that it influences how others see individuals who need or use AAC.

In recent years, the general public has become somewhat better informed about the extreme situation of people with the locked-in syndrome. The movie "The Diving Bell and the Butterfly" has made a strong impression on the public and has contributed to raising awareness everywhere of the dramatic impact of the loss of communication on a person's life.

Individuals who recover after a severe loss of language and communication occasionally report how frightening the experience is. Hamilton Cameron (cited in Lebrun, 1978, p. 50) reported that he went through feelings of terror when, one morning, he woke up in a state of hemiplegia and speechlessness. He had suffered a cerebral thrombosis during the night. "It was about seven o'clock . . . when I awakened. I had no sensation of pain. I simply awakened and came to the realization that during the night I suffered a paralytic aphasic stroke. I could not talk. I was immovable, and I had a fantastic sensation of being enveloped in a leather bag molded to my body. Then came a radical sensation of torturous fear, an almost indefinable sense of terror. I was in agony in my despair. I was a prey to the incubus of impending death."

But not every AAC condition is as severe as the locked-in syndrome. One of the basic principles of communication (on which AAC is built) is that there is always communication. The purpose of AAC is to find the best possible adaptations to make communication as effective and satisfactory as possible. We know that this is, unfortunately, a goal that is only seldom reached. Communication is not always realized to its fullest extent and, despite all the attempts of users, caregivers, friends, and others—frustration, misunderstandings, loneliness, anger, and feeling of incompleteness sometimes look like being intrinsic parts of life for an AAC user. Realizing that you know what you want to say and being unable to express yourself brings serious frustration. We know from studies of the social-emotional condition of aphasia that anger is often part of this frustration.

In recent years, interest in the unique and intriguing experience of AAC users (and their partners) has arisen. In a 2010 episode of the popular series "Law and Order/Special Victims Unit," the team tries to help a nonspeaking woman to communicate to identify her rapist (Black, 2010). Rummel-Hudson's touching real-life story about his nonspeaking daughter (Rummel-Hudson, 2008), and Draper's fictitious story (Draper, 2012) about a young girl named Melody, written for a young public of readers show both a growing fascination for the uniqueness of the AAC experience.

THE UNIQUENESS OF THE AAC EXPERIENCE

It is hard—and probably impossible—for a person who is not an AAC user to fully understand the breath of "the AAC experience." AAC users feel the need to "compare notes" with other AAC users, to get ideas about how others cope with the daily experience of being misunderstood (by many) and being socially and cognitively underestimated because one is not fast or precise enough in expressing an opinion or in coming up with a sharp reply.

Bryen, Chung, and Seagalman (2009) discuss the prevalence of depression and social isolation in individuals who are AAC users. They looked at postings through the electronic listserve for AAC users (see further in this chapter) and spotted a high number of personal disclosures such as, "I have depression and considered taking my life," "not being able to do anything for myself makes me want to die," and "even though I have a smile on my face every day does not mean I don't get lonely and depressed." Based on their observations and experience, the authors report that electronic networking for AAC users can reduce social isolation and loneliness. The electronic community can "provide a platform for counseling and social/emotional support."

Michael Williams started an e-mail-mentoring group for young AAC users in 1998. Through e-mail, Williams and his collaborators paired young AAC users with AAC users with a lot of experience. The rationale came down to: "Disabled individuals with several years of disability experience are frequently better aware of the needs of disabled people and better informed about government benefits than able-bodied professionals in the rehabilitation delivery system" (p. 285). Individuals who are AAC users share a unique situation that may not be entirely understood by non-AAC users. Typically developing children and adolescents, as well as adults, continuously learn strategies to cope with a variety of mundane and profound issues: how to make friends, how to fall in love, how to negotiate, how to combine work and family, how to plan for a vacation, how to budget, how to be witty and silly, how to be appropriate (and how to be inappropriate), how to plan for a career, how to shop for a car, how to find out how sexuality works, how to stay out of trouble, how to brag, how to talk about your parents (and show your exasperation), how to hang out with your friends, and more. Several mentoring networks and organizations have grown in spontaneous ways, most often initiated by people

who are AAC users. One example is Chris Klein who has set up the mentoring and education AAC network service by and for individuals who need support in discovering their own talents as AAC users (http://www.becomeaac.com/home).

A COMMUNITY OF AAC USERS

For almost all activities and events of life, nondisabled people have models around them (not to mention movies and TV) that give ideas about how things are done. But where do AAC users look to know how these things are done by an AAC user? Other AAC users may be the best models and mentors.

That is one reason why communities of AAC users have emerged, with the sole purpose of interacting with each other. Already during special youth camps for young AAC users, this is obvious. In 1999, I was invited by Joan Bruno to visit Camp Chatterbox, a summer camp in New Jersey for children who use AAC. Everything in the camp is built around the experience and learning-for-life by the AAC users, their parents, and their caregivers (in that order, yes). Joan has been running this camp with a group of enthusiastic volunteers since 1992. The same children often return each year to participate again in the camp. That should not surprise us because there is so much to learn for AAC users just by observing other AAC users. It makes you wonder: from which do the children and adolescents learn most, from the activities that have been programmed or just from the fact that there are so many AAC users together who are an inspiration for one another? Similar camps are now run during the summer in several locations in the United States and elsewhere.

More then two decades ago, Bryen (2008) and her collaborators at Temple University started a listserve for AAC users: ACOLUG, which stands for Augmentative Communication Online Users Group. This listserve attempts to "provide a forum for AAC users to connect, support, and learn from each other." Years and years of intensive daily e-mail communications by 700 subscribers make for an impressive archive of discussion about small and big things in the lives of individuals who use AAC. Reading through these messages, one easily comes to the realization how much the "AAC condition" permeates a person's entire life. Let's look at a few examples:

Where Do I Get Help?

This is a common theme that comes back again and again. Understandably, the world of AAC users has many specifics that outsiders don't know about. What are my chances to get accepted in my community? How do I deal with all kinds of administrative or other bumps in the road? Newcomers, often parents of young children who are new AAC users, are desperately trying to find their way in the complex world of AAC devices, helping professionals agencies, manufacturers and vendors, insurance companies, and Medicaid. AAC users, or parents with several years of experience under their belt, can help newcomers and direct them to parent groups that will help them deal with questions and ideas for IEPs and other issues. A recurring theme is, "Now that I have the device, who will help me figure out how it works and how can I use it to its maximum potential?" For example: "I taught myself (AAC device operating system) by pressing buttons. I am amazed

how many people get (manufacturing company name) devices without having a support behind them. I don't understand why (manufacturing company name) is so popular without a better support."

Discussions About What Works Best

"I use scanning as a selection technique, but now I have met students who have been discouraged from looking for employment because of their selection method." Answer from an AAC user: "That is ridiculous—I have been scanning for over 21 years, went to college for a creative writing degree, and have two jobs now. Sure, let me talk to them!"

The Broken AAC Device

"My (name of device) was back at (name of the device manufacturing company) for 6 weeks. I got a loaner, which worked ok, but I waited for my own device. When it finally came, it was acting sluggish, and the screen is getting harder to push. I don't know whether I should send it back or keep it and learn how to deal with the problems. I don't have much respect for (name of the manufacturing company)'s quality."

The New and Better AAC Device—Or Not So Much Better

There is obviously a segment of the AAC population that closely follows the developments in AAC technology. Will the new model of (name of company) be much better? I heard there are problems with the interface? It is easy to see why many AAC users are investing time and energy in following the AAC technology. Better technology, so it is implicitly hoped, means better quality of life. Short messages like, "I can't wait to get my new device," and "Well, more good news. I am so excited I won't sleep all weekend now. They shipped it out yesterday I think, and it will be here this Monday!" are very common.

Reading the hundreds of postings discussing the challenges, choices, and sometimes the joy of having a communication device, makes it clear that the device does play a powerful role in the life of the user. And this is not to be compared with the obsession of the sports car fan or the baseball nut who wants to have and discuss all the gadgets or discuss the pros and cons of sport cars or baseball. These are discussions about something that is the lifeline for many—these are not trivial discussions. Most AAC users understand all too well that their quality of life, their ability to connect to others, their personal future, and possibly their hope of a career depends on good communication solutions.

Sexuality

Individuals with disabilities face the same challenges as able-bodied people. Everybody seeks happiness, social contact, self-realizations, and respect from others. Communication is vital in pursuing these objectives in everyone's life. Sexuality can be at the same time a unique way of self-expression and reaching togetherness with a loved partner. However, parents and educators often feel insecure and awkward thinking of or addressing these areas of life. Many feel ambiguous about including words and concepts that refer to sexuality in AAC vocabulary. In their discussion groups, AAC users argue back

and forth whether the right to sexuality should get more attention during conferences, research, and most importantly, throughout their life.

AAC AS A NORMAL PHENOMENON

I have argued that the AAC device in our society should become as accepted and even unnoticed as a pair of eyeglasses, and in some way as accepted as the use of a wheelchair. In a not so distant past, people stared at individuals who were pushed by others around in a wheelchair. People with severe mobility limitations simply were not expected to move around in public areas. It was an uncommon sight. Emancipation movements by groups of individuals with disabilities worldwide and their advocates have changed this scene. In the streets of the cities, in trains, in restaurants, churches, and all public places today, individuals who are in wheelchairs have, fortunately, become a common sight. Their participation in community activities is evident and healthy for all members of the community. It is to be hoped that the use of AAC will also become a common phenomenon, and that it will allow all members of society to welcome everyone and enjoy the richness and diversity in how things are done and how individuals communicate.

POINTS TO REMEMBER

- Being an AAC user is, for many, a unique condition of life that has an influence on a person's perception of identity and, in many cases, the way a person's identity is seen by others.

- Artistic expressions in poetry, visual arts, and films have been and continue to be useful attempts to express the uniqueness and dignity of people who use AAC.
- The community of AAC users functions as a network that allows communication and interaction. A network of connections exists that helps with information exchange, mentoring, social and emotional support, and education.
- The more society considers AAC as a phenomenon within the normal range of varieties in which people express themselves and interact with the world, the more likely it becomes that AAC users will be full participants in community life.

REFERENCES

Black, P. (Director). (2010). *Law & order: Special victims unit: Disabled* (Season 11, Episode 17) [Video/DVD].

Bryen, D. (2008). *ACOLUG—Augmentative communication online users' group.* Presentation at the International Society for Augmentative and Alternative Communication conference, Montreal, Canada.

Bryen, D., Chung, Y., & Segalman, B. (2009). Depression, social isolation, and ACOLUG. In P. Formica, R. Conti, & S. Osgood (Eds.), *Proceedings of the Biennial Pittsburgh Employment Conference for Augmented Communicators* (pp. 13–20). Pittsburgh, PA: SHOUT Press.

Draper, S. (2012). *Out of my mind.* New York, NY: Atheneum Books for Young Readers.

Folkins, J. (2013). *Resource on person-first language.* Retrieved from http://www.asha.org/publications/journals/submissions/person_first.htm

Klein, C. (2013). *Becomeaac.* Retrieved from http://www.becomeaac.com/home

Lebrun, Y. (1978). The inside of aphasia. In Y. Lebrun & R. Hoops (Eds.), *The management of aphasia* (pp. 50–55). Lisse, the Netherlands: Swets & Zeitlinger.

Rummel-Hudson, R. (2008). *Schuyler's monster. A father's journey with his wordless daughter.* New York, NY: St. Martin's Griffin.

Williams, M., & Krezman, C. (Eds.). (2000). *Beneath the surface: Creative expressions of augmented communicators* (ISAAC Series: Vol. 2 ed.). Toronto, Canada: International Society for Augmentative and Alternative Communication.

Index